The Intensivist's Challenge

David Crippen

Editor

The Intensivist's Challenge

Aging and Career Growth in a High-Stress Medical Specialty

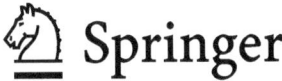 Springer

Editor
David Crippen
Department of Critical Care Medicine
University of Pittsburgh
Pittsburgh, PA
USA

ISBN 978-3-319-30452-6   ISBN 978-3-319-30454-0   (eBook)
DOI 10.1007/978-3-319-30454-0

Library of Congress Control Number: 2016938432

Printed on acid-free paper

This Springer imprint is published by Springer Nature
The registered company is Springer International Publishing AG Switzerland

Foreword

I still read the odd journal that comes in the mail, and through the electronic waterfalls. In this week's selection, there seemed to be a number of articles written by people, with whom I podiumed over the years, who were older than me. "Still charging the windmills" I thought. And there were some advertisements for industry functions spruiking some unfathomable device to measure blood flow starring some of the usual suspects. But many of the names who shared my journey are vanishing.

The real pioneers have been slowly vanishing for some time. The baby boomers represent the second echelon. It was they who turned the inspiration of the Safars, Thompsons, Civettas, Shoemakers, Rapins, Grenviks, and Bursteins into a functional specialty. And now their time has come to go gently into the night.

Intensive and Critical Care, like other specialties, have a number of unique features. Not least of these is that it has been an emerging specialty. It has been established for many years that the sickest patients are best looked after together in a special place, and in most countries, it is recognized that they are best cared for by specialist doctors and nurses. Successful intensive care seems to be dependent upon specialist presence at the bedside and the building of teams consisting of people who are empowered and entrusted. The toys are very seductive, although they are becoming very much more complex. Those I know who loved their careers in intensive care were those who valued the outrageous privilege of being invited into the personal space of patients and families in crisis. Many were my mentors and friends: our paths ran together for variable periods. Those interactions are among my best memories. For people such as these, leaving what was their second home is a wrench. I did badly initially.

Aging practitioners are affected by a number of sensory and cognitive changes including declining processing speed, reduced problem-solving ability, reduced manual dexterity, deteriorating hearing and sight, and the introduction to the risks of aging. And yet, there is an increasing tendency to get rid of compulsory retirement age as we recognize the great variation in competence and the value of wisdom and experience. When I teach students, I supervise their self-motivated and self-run learning. I am there to keep them on the track. I think my value is to add to what they have gleaned from papers and text, both in perspective and relevance. I think I do this through experience and hopefully wisdom largely through patient stories. I have a lot of the latter.

Someone said to me once, "if people are prepared to give you money for doing something you love doing, and you are doing it well, why would you stop?" Why are many of my senior colleagues still spruiking and writing, and why am I not?

How do you know when the time has come to go? It may be driven by health problems or frustration at the ever-increasing difficulty of dealing with the bureaucracy. A reduction in clinical hours means a reduction in the procedural aspects and some, particularly insertion of intra-aortic balloons, require rigid following the sequence to ensure the correct placement and safety. For me the messages began with some health problems, but it was realizing that I was no longer wanting to get out of bed to meet the needs of others that ultimately put me into a nonclinical role.

And yet leaving your second home after many years is not an easy path, no matter how well prepared you think you are. When the time came, we had enough money. We had saved up for our old age although learning to spend it has been part of the adaption. But perhaps the most important thing about moving into retirement for me is not something I have read in any book. When you have worked, as I did, in a job that you loved for over 30 years, you find that few of the problems you encountered outside that job become a significant deterrent to happiness. When you take away the consuming passion, they acquire a new significance. I miss the team and the families but don't seem to miss the patients. Although I love it, past patients stop me in the street to tell me how wonderful I used to be.

Most of the authors in this book are known to me. It appears, although I am not sure, that they are mostly still working. One might wonder at their credibility to write about their future journey. This book demands a second edition in 5 years to see how they went. It was not what I thought.

What do I do now? A bit of medical stuff, a committee I value (having ditched most of those I initially joined, some teaching, some charity work, and an assistant tour guide at a museum of mechanical music. I help older people off and on merry-go-rounds. I think of myself as a geriatric Catcher in the Rye. I go to a gym and play bowls. Which I will get back to after tomorrow's arthroscopy. I take my pills.

You see, there is much to learn about the new journey that is not in anything I read.

There are a lot of funerals to attend. Once a month a group of peers and colleagues and I meet for lunch because we only saw each other at funerals. As De Niro says in "The Intern," there are a lot of funerals.

I still have a little to do with my old unit. The Golden Rule is that you have no unsolicited opinions about the job you left and only good opinions of your successors.

I have learned to travel without slides (or a USB), and it is a better alternative. One big change is that my current partner (of 50 years) spends more in toyshops than art galleries.

I am re-engaging with locals and people you have lost contact with and trying to stay in touch with people you value. But now the conversation in clubs and bars and at dinner tables may be about golf, grandchildren, or investment as opposed to patients and health care.

I remember Hammarskoldt's admonition that loneliness is not having no one to tell your troubles to but about having no one to telling you their troubles. Be altruistic. Not just through charities but have a few individuals to help.

I try to eat healthy. If you are into evidence-based medicine, don't even try to determine what sort of food is best for you. What it all boils down to really is that fruit and vegetables are better than red meat and hamburgers. And one glass a day is good for you. I have an obsolescence plan for the wine cellar, so it will be nearly empty when I reach my actuarially calculated demise date (from which I have taken off 8 years for bad behavior.)

I have a Will, an enduring power of attorney, and an advance care plan which names a person responsible for decision making.

Enjoy family. And stay in touch with old friends.

Most of the above I doubt will make the chapters that follow. They were part of a difficult learning curve when I embraced a new life and a new journey very different from the old. I am enjoying it now. But I am still looking for a last windmill to charge. Although I am devoid of any political activity like Arnie, "I will return." Perhaps.

Sydney, NSW, Australia   Malcolm Fisher, AO, MBChB, MD, FCICM, FRCA

Introduction: The Senior Intensivist and the Aging Brain

"People try to put us d-down
Just because we get around
Things they do look awful c-c-cold
I hope I die before I get old"

The Who, "My Generation," 1965

This volume is a treatise on the inevitabilities of aging for acute care physicians. What are the options for these physicians when they either choose to quit working, having grown tired of it, or are pushed out for various reasons, sometimes to make room for younger entrants, sometimes because brain fade makes it difficult to keep up with the increasingly complex science?

The reality of life is that we're born, we live for a while, we get old, and then we die. The hallmark of our lives is how we live in the time we have available to us and, in today's culture of aging gracefully, how we order our career exit. The unanswered question is: Do we slow down and deteriorate because of generalized social privation during aging, or do we suffer some gentle form of brain failure?

Many things have changed in the new millennium that affect our longevity. In the early 1960s, the average life expectancy in the United States was 70.2 years. In 2013, the average life expectancy was 78.8 years [1]. However, the quality of life of aging Americans has not increased commensurately. In the 1960s, the incidence of dementia among people approaching death was less than 1 %. Currently, the incidence of dementia in Americans is between 5 and 7 % for adults age 60 or older. Starting at age 65, the risk of developing some form of dementia doubles every 5 years. By age 85 years, between 25 % and 50 % of people will exhibit signs of Alzheimer's disease [2]. We are living longer, but despite rapid advances in health care, we are less interactive.

The issue of subtle, age-related deterioration of brain function is difficult to sort out. The "heart too good to die" concept as espoused by Peter Safar does not apply to the brain [3]. The brain is a rather frail organ, rapidly damaged during hemodynamic or metabolic disasters and difficult to resuscitate. The heart is relatively easy to restart by traditional CPR. The brain has proven to be dramatically less so [4].

How do progressive physiological changes in brain function affect the choices intensivists face in their emeritus years?

Progressive brain insufficiency invariably affects consciousness on many levels. Consciousness is structurally produced in the cerebral hemispheres, including the pons and the medulla. These structures are all interconnected by the reticular formation, which begins in the medulla and extends to the midbrain, where it forms the reticular activating system. This pathway modulates the perception of events and controls integrated responses [5]. A common axiom was that the average brain loses about 10,000 brain cells a day by attrition. But there are more than 100 billion neurons in the typical human brain [6], so even a loss of 10,000 neurons per day would seem to contribute little to this deterioration.

Cerebral atrophy occurs naturally in aging and is accelerated between the ages of 70 and 90. But the process actually begins subclinically in the gray matter of the cerebral cortex at a much earlier age [7]. The average gray matter volume decreases from about 390 mL at age 22 to about 300 mL at age 82 [8]. Total brain mass loss between the ages of 20 and 80 is around 450 g, or roughly one-third of the previous brain volume, assuming no new disease process such as Alzheimer's [9]. Although the exact physiological process continues to be somewhat controversial, we do know that cerebral atrophy is global, relentless, and functionally pathological.

Gray matter is where most cerebral processing takes place, so cellular loss should affect our ability to accurately and quickly solve problems [7]. Part of the chores of repeating routine daily tasks such as dressing, eating breakfast, and driving to work may be affected with age by deterioration of connections between gray and white matter neurons. Specific areas of the brain seem to degenerate at different rates. It is unclear whether "normal" cerebral atrophy during aging affects each brain the same way or how each cognitive area is affected [10], and loss of brain volume does not necessarily equate to loss of brain cells. The number of cells may not change, but their volume and character can definitely increase and decrease, much like skeletal muscle cells.

Cognitive abilities such as verbal fluency increase until the mid-50s but start to deteriorate in the sixth decade, after which most of the neocortex continues to degenerate until death [11]. Some experts suggest that cerebral atrophy correlates with recall deficits during cognitive testing in aging patients [12]. Many people in their fifth and sixth decades experience "word searching" and a transient inability to recall previously known names. This variety of cognitive deterioration is associated with hippocampal inadequacy.

Unfortunately, it does not appear that the brain has much of any intrinsic capability for cellular repair or replacement, so we're left with what we're left with. However, this neurological degradation can be camouflaged somewhat by several compensatory mechanisms, including denial and frustration. More to the point, aging people trade cognitive decline for enhanced judgment. As processing speed slows in late life, logic, reasoning, and spatial abilities remain generally well preserved. Older individuals' life experience, their long accumulation of knowledge, and their maturity and wisdom offset some of the losses in processing capability.

The difference between categorical knowledge and wisdom might be explained this way: An adult tells a child to play in their safe yard and not in traffic. The child has the *knowledge* and ability to play anywhere but lacks the *wisdom* to refrain from dangerous behavior [13].

The issue of enhanced maturity comes quickly into play in the aging intensivist. It can be argued that reduced processing speed, short-term memory loss, and difficulty keeping abreast of rapidly changing knowledge can effectively be traded for mature judgment, life experience, and ability to teach.

Therapies for the vicissitudes of the aging brain are years away from practical application. When these treatments do become clinically available (and FDA approved), they will likely be used first for patients with other life-threatening diseases, such as Huntington's disease or amyotrophic lateral sclerosis, not for persons with simply slowing, aging brains.

There is, however, hope for the future. Extensive research is being performed regarding cognitive function (and deterioration) in the aging brain. The "Salt Cognitive Aging Laboratory" at the University of Virginia is conducting active, longitudinal studies of aging in patients from ages 18–98 years [14]. These studies include a thorough initial assessment followed by several follow-ups. The data from this project have yielded a substantial knowledge base [15].

So thereby hangs much of the dilemma of aging for high-end patient care providers. The fires in the belly do burn down to embers in time. Is the burning-down process social, with the intensivist simply "getting tired" over a period of years and losing interest? Or is there a component of brain failure involved? Is there a place for the teaching of the strong suit of aging—that is, judgment? Is this judgment desired in an otherwise technological specialty? Is someone willing to pay for accessing it? Some of these questions are explored in this volume.

Pittsburgh, PA, USA   David Crippen, MD, FCCM

References

1. U.S. Department of Health and Human Services, Administration for Community Living: Administration on Aging (AoA): The Older Population. Available at: http://www.aoa.acl.gov/ Aging_Statistics/Profile/2014/3.aspx.
2. Crippen D. Brain failure and brain death. In: Souba WW, Fink MP, Jurkovich GJ, et al., editors. ACS surgery: principles & practice. 6th ed. New York: WebMD; 2007. p. 1609–11.
3. American Speech-Language-Hearing Association: Dementia. Available at: http://www.asha. org/PRPSpecificTopic.aspx?folderid=8589935289&section=Incidence_and_Prevalence.
4. Brindley PG, Markland DM, Mayers I, et al. Predictors of survival following in-hospital adult cardiopulmonary resuscitation. CMAJ. 2002;167:343–8.
5. Pinault D. The thalamic reticular nucleus: structure, function and concept. Brain Res Brain Res Rev. 2004;46:1–31.
6. Pakkenberg B, Gundersen HJG. Neocortical neuron number in humans: effect of sex and age. J Comp Neurol. 1997;384:312–20.

7. Hedden T, Gabrieli JD. Insights into the aging mind: a view from cognitive neuroscience. Nat Rev Neurosci. 2004;5:87–96, 14735112.

8. Courchesne E, Chisum HJ, Townsend J, et al. Normal brain development and aging: quantitative analysis at in vivo MR imaging in healthy volunteers. Radiology. 2000;216:672–82.

9. Franke K, Ziegler G, Klöppel S, et al. Alzheimer's Disease Neuroimaging Initiative: Estimating the age of healthy subjects from T1-weighted MRI scans using kernel methods: exploring the influence of various parameters. Neuroimage. 2010;50:883–92, 20070949.

10. Burgmans S, van Boxtel MP, Vuurman EF, et al. The prevalence of cortical gray matter atrophy may be overestimated in the healthy aging brain. Neuropsychology. 2009;23:541–50.

11. Schaie KW. Intellectual development in adulthood: the Seattle Longitudinal Study. Cambridge, UK/New York: Cambridge University Press; 1996.

12. Yassa MA, Muftuler LT, Starka CEL, et al. Ultrahigh-resolution microstructural diffusion tensor imaging reveals perforant path degradation in aged humans in vivo. Proc Natl Acad Sci U S A. 2010;107:12687–91.

13. Darwin M. The urgent need for a brain centered approach to geroprotection for cryonicists. Chronosphere (blog). 2001. Available at: http://chronopause.com/chronopause.com/index.php/2011/05/31/going-going-gone...-part-2/.

14. Cognitive Aging Laboratory: Research in the Cognitive Aging Laboratory. Available at: http://faculty.virginia.edu/cogage/.

15. Cognitive Aging Laboratory: Resources. Available at: http://faculty.virginia.edu/cogage/links/publications/.

Contents

Contributors

Marie R. Baldisseri Department of Critical Care Medicine, University of Pittsburgh Medical Center, Pittsburgh, PA, USA

Thomas P. Bleck Neurological Sciences, Rush Medical College, Chicago, IL, USA

Clinical Neurophysiology, Rush University Medical Center, Chicago, IL, USA

Richard Burrows Private Practice, Bon Secours Hospital, Galway, Ireland

Donald B. Chalfin Jefferson College of Population Health of Thomas Jefferson University, Philadelphia, PA, USA

David Crippen Department of Critical Care Medicine, University of Pittsburgh Medical Center, Pittsburgh, PA, USA

Ake Grenvik Department of Critical Care Medicine, University of Pittsburgh Medical Center, Pittsburgh, PA, USA

Ross Hofmeyr Department of Anaesthesia and Perioperative Medicine, Faculty of Health Sciences, University of Cape Town, Cape Town, South Africa

John W. Hoyt Pittsburgh Critical Care Associates, Inc., Pittsburgh, PA, USA

Critical Care Medicine, University of Pittsburgh Medical Center, Pittsburgh, PA, USA

W. Andrew Kofke Department of Anesthesiology and Critical Care, University of Pennsylvania, Philadelphia, PA, USA

Guy Kositratna Department of Anesthesiology and Critical Care, University of Pennsylvania, Philadelphia, PA, USA

Joseph Lex Department of Emergency Medicine, Temple University School of Medicine, Philadelphia, PA, USA

Mark A. Mazer Department of Critical Care Medicine, Vidant Medical Center, Greenville, NC, USA

Brad Power Department of Intensive Care, Sir Charles Gairdner Hospital, Perth, WA, Australia

James V. Snyder Critical Care Medicine, University of Pittsburgh Medical Center, Pittsburgh, PA, USA

Stephen Streat Department of Critical Care Medicine, Auckland City Hospital, Grafton, Auckland, New Zealand

Errington C. Thompson Department of Surgery, Marshall University, Huntington, WV, USA

Brian Wowk 21st Century Medicine, Inc., Fontana, CA, USA

Chapter 1
"Fire in the Belly": Youth and Exuberance

David Crippen

> *"Ah, but I was so much older then.*
> *I'm younger than that now".*

Bob Dylan. My back pages. 1964.

> *"Traveling eternity road*
> *What will you find there?*
> *Carrying your heavy load*
> *Searching to find a piece of mind"*

The Moody Blues, "Eternity Road," 1969

Prologue

At age 70, I was a master of the universe. I was riding a motorcycle up the Adriatic coast and playing guitar in a rock band at the House of Blues in New Orleans. I thought I would live and work forever, or until I was found dead slumped in a nurses' station somewhere. Then, in a few seconds, it all changed. Some of this change was due to bad luck and bad timing, but most of it was due, ultimately, to age.

What follows is a chronicle of this saga, written in the first person. I have lumped some similar facts into smaller bites and glossed over others to make the narrative more readable. I describe the rise, the crest, and the decline and then analyze the options available to me and how I managed to find something meaningful from them. Hopefully there is something of value here for others facing similar situations.

In the Beginning, There Was… Me

When I was a younger dog, the road to my goal was very clear and precise. I had visions of what I wanted to do and where I wanted to go and a pretty good idea of what it would take to get there. The devil was in the details. Few faced more

D. Crippen, MD, FCCM
Department of Critical Care Medicine, University of Pittsburgh Medical Center,
644a Scaife Hall, Pittsburgh, PA 15261, USA
e-mail: crippen@pitt.edu

© Springer International Publishing Switzerland 2016
D. Crippen (ed.), *The Intensivist's Challenge: Aging and Career Growth in a High-Stress Medical Specialty*, DOI 10.1007/978-3-319-30454-0_1

obstacles to a career in medicine than I did. I stayed on that path with perseverance and stubborn determination, enduring trial and error shunts along the way.

In what passed for an academic system in the early 1960s, there were three desirable classifications of kids in high school: jocks (for whom grades were not a consideration), National Honor Society members, and class clowns. Jocks went on to teach physical education in high schools, NHS members went on to big colleges and did their parents proud, and class clowns went on to become Richard Pryor. The educational system lost interest in everyone else and labeled them as not amenable to education.

The teachers applied themselves only to the kids who fit the stereotype of a desirable student. I was an outlier, and therefore I was surely defective. The school counselor told my father I was borderline "retarded," and his best bet would be to get me out with a diploma if possible and get me into the army quickly so I wouldn't be a financial drain on him. I was in the bottom quarter of my high school graduating class. My father encouraged me to just do what I could and make the best of it. Not much was expected.

But even though the college system was unimpressed with my overall record, my SAT scores were just high enough that the state university had to accept me, and I was admitted to the university on academic probation in 1962. Predictably, not having a clue about how to study or to absorb information as presented at the school, I flunked classes. My average grade overall was well below a C.

About this time, the US Army started looking for candidates to protect the world from the creeping ravages of communism in Southeast Asia. Dodging the draft was difficult for those with grades like mine, but a cottage industry of small colleges willing to accept any student with financial means sprang up, and I remained safe for a while nestled in one. My ilk came from all over the country: we had flunked out or busted out of colleges everywhere, and none of us were ever expected to be anything other than a burden to our families.

I was trying, but I had no idea how to study and had learned nothing in any previous schooling. I promptly flunked again, which brought my cumulative average down to 1.9, and there was an army Jeep waiting for me at the end of the sidewalk. I was drafted in the summer of 1967, and my college career was over.

The Jeep at the End of My Path

I was 24 years old, and my resume included flunking out of two colleges and working a motley assortment of minimum-wage jobs. I was looking at failure from the inside out. The military was the end of the line for losers, and I was a loser of the first order. Since there was nothing left but the military, I entered the army like a lamb. The army was less than impressed with me, and I was made a combat medic, one minor step up from rifleman. I figured out quickly that the army was going to be a tough gig, one that would probably end with my name on a wall somewhere. I wound up in Vietnam as a field (para)medic, serving there from 1968 to early 1970.

The military and Vietnam cleaned up my act dramatically, teaching me responsibility and discipline, which I could never have learned elsewhere. I became a radically different person. Sometime between 1968 and 1969, I received my calling in a very Howard Beale-like apocalypse: a flash of lightning, a clap of thunder, and a stone at my feet that read "doctor." Like Howard Beale, I followed this calling meekly to its furthest extent, knowing that I would suffer but that in the end, my goal would be fulfilled.

Fire in My Belly

I will spare you the details, but I really did make deals with God in exchange for my life somewhere in the A Shau Valley. You don't really understand the concept of God until you start making deals with him when your life is flashing before your eyes. My part of the bargain was simply to do the best I could for people. God came through: every time a door slammed shut in my face, another opened. I do not believe this was accidental. No one in the universe had less likelihood of arriving where I am than I. It is impossible that my path was a series of random events.

I wanted to be a doctor more than anything in the world. I thought of nothing else. I steamrollered every obstacle and never let go of my goal for an instant. When I fell, I got up. When I fell again, I got up again. I saw the sunrise as I studied stupid things I knew I would never see again. I read volumes of back issues of *Time* to improve my score on the MCAT. There was *nothing* I would have not done to get where I am. Idiot bureaucrats, gatekeepers, managers, and geeky, suit-clad administrators didn't faze me; their roadblocks didn't matter. The passion encompassed all.

One of the most potent incentives to achieve success is failure. I believe that part of what has gotten me through is the fact that I know failure intimately. I have failed in my life on occasion, and I have looked a bleak future in the face. I've had to cope with disappointments, and setbacks and disheartenment, and pain and people that threatened to end it all. I've experienced times when success was so close and yet so far. But I also know the feeling of wanting something so intensely that I'd do anything to get it—and that there was no power in heaven or earth that could stop me.

Similarly, I clawed my way to the top of the academic heap (more or less) as a resident and eventually an attending physician in critical care. Equal portions of dumb luck and being in the right place at the right time propelled me along.

Theater of the Invalid

As I aged, the inevitable fall from grace seemed to be far enough away as to not be particularly noticeable. My professional and personal life bloomed, with no sign of wilting. I thought I would live and prosper forever. Then a sudden, unpredicted, unexpected physical decompensation in this otherwise healthy, active 69-year-old physician set me on the road that brought me here.

In November 2012, I developed convincing but mild symptoms of Guillain-Barré syndrome a week after a routine influenza vaccine injection. These passed quickly and my condition was not treated with anything other than continued observation. Then in April 2015, I developed sudden onset of weakness in the right arm and left lower extremity and landed in the emergency department, where dozens of scans and tests were done. All findings were either normal or not remarkably different from those in 2012. Then I progressed to becoming quadriparetic with no bladder or bowel function. I could do virtually nothing for myself, but mercifully there was no respiratory compromise.

I then had an EMG, which compared to the previous one was markedly more abnormal. Therefore, the working diagnosis continued to be a variant of Guillain-Barré syndrome. Ultimately I received 5 days of intravenous IgG, following which I did improve somewhat. I moved from wheelchair to walker to cane over about 8 months, although as I sit and write this, I am still limited to fairly short walking distances. It is unclear whether my condition will ever return to baseline.

I will add here that during admission for short-term inpatient rehabilitation, I was asked if I wanted to attend a support group (for debilitated patients). I said yes, having little else to do. It turned out to be a very Catholic prayer group, and I was the infidel salmon that leapt out of the suds onto the shore. About ten denizens of the spinal rehab unit attended, all devout Catholics, as this was a Catholic hospital. Most were in motorized wheelchairs, many had multiple other medical problems, and all were in terrible physical condition, sustained by "medical miracles" that wrestled the Reaper from the bedside but did little to maintain much quality of life.

Ultimately, the time came for individual prayers (I, the failed Baptist, faked it with generic platitudes). Without exception, each of them thanked God that their infirmities were not any worse and expressed hope for those in worse shape. I was moved to tears.

My indolent and debilitating situation played havoc with my clinical schedule, forcing others to stand in for me in various capacities. As the months passed, it became obvious that continuation of my career as it had been was open to question.

Barbarians at the Gate

I was 71 years of age, and it dawned on me that younger physicians were being actively recruited to fulfill roles in my department, roles that had evolved away from what they were 30 years previously. My areas of expertise had moved away from understanding and interpreting the evolving science to the use of clinical judgment and intuition based on 30 years' experience. It was now uncertain whether I could do both. The practice of medicine was radically evolving, and I wasn't evolving well with it.

The science of critical care had changed its focus from clinical intuition to expanding technology. I practiced medicine from a visceral vantage. I used my intuition and all my senses to sort out patient care issues, relegating "tests" to confirmation of what I already knew. I could look at patients at the bedside and sense a great deal of what their problems were. All that was being replaced by many different alternatives.

Medical school was radically changing. In the clinical years of medical school in the 1970s, I was the first to arrive at the hospital and the last to leave. I had patient care responsibility and I was expected to take care of the patients. I was responsible for something important, and if I couldn't or wouldn't do it, I got my butt kicked by a chief resident. Medical students now get more lectures, book learning, and simulation centers. They complain if they feel they have too much work and it interferes with their lives [1].

I endured every-other-night hospital call during my surgery residency program at Bellevue, every third night in my critical care fellowship at Pitt. I saw everything, learned most of it, and also learned to survive and efficiently deal with an overwhelming workload. Those who couldn't or wouldn't were let go or transferred to a lighter-load program. The rigorous programs selected for the most aggressive, committed residents, and I was one. We'd seen it all and nothing surprised us in clinical medicine, even (especially?) at three in the morning.

All these features are becoming discredited now as abusive. Today's medical students get into medical school on high grades and savvy about how to make themselves look good on their curricula vitae. If they learn anything on rounds, it's from the back row, and if they complain they're overworked, the institution must lighten their schedules.

Soulless technology upstages physical medicine. Modern residents and fellows are learning that nothing can be trusted unless they can see it on echo, MRI, or a computer screen. In so doing, they're losing the ability to actually see and feel patients. Residents and fellows also complain if they think they're overworked. Direct patient care is being taken over by mid-level providers: physician's assistants and nurse practitioners. Robots with TV screens are examining patients for providers miles away. I fear for the future. I am the last of my kind.

Dangerous Choices

Eventually and inevitably, a close physician friend in my department with a high clinical administrative role asked to see me in my office. He diplomatically suggested that I consider looking out from my blinders to see whether there might be another career option beckoning. Perhaps I had reached the point of no return in a world that had passed many of my previous talents (and opinions) by. Perhaps the time had come to consider where my strengths and weaknesses lay in this new world.

As a practical matter, my department owed me nothing. I had been a (seemingly) valuable part of it for 15 years, and it was time for me to retire in some fashion, if for no other reason than to make room for newcomers entering a small club. The department could have simply organized a farewell party and bid me good luck in my future.

Had that occurred, I would have been in serious psychiatric trouble. Medicine for me was not a job; it defined my life, and I had no concept of "retirement" (a term used to describe the killing of replicants in 1982's *Blade Runner*). Medicine was my entire life, and without it, my entire being would collapse. I had beaten myself to a pulp and endured every possible hardship to get where I was, and I thought I could do it till they found me collapsed and dead, over a computer terminal somewhere in an ICU. I thought I would live forever and work forever.

There is a dangerous precedent for these issues of "retirement" in highly committed people if they get stuck in the past.

In his prime, novelist and essayist Hunter S. Thompson was brilliant, insightful, and unpredictable [2, 3]. He absorbed and then described the world of the 1960s and 1970s spontaneously and with a unique quirkiness, a radically new concept in writing. He viewed history and he made history.

As he matured, the world matured on a separate axis. As age took its toll, he ran out of capacity and life just wasn't fun anymore. In 2005, at the age of 67, Thompson was found dead of a self-inflicted gunshot wound. He had considered his life a perfection that simply ran its course. Failure and mediocrity were unacceptable to him, and his basic nature would not allow evolution to emeritus status. He chose to exit before he reached the bottom.

As it turned out, the door I had never noticed before opened, and I had the ability to see the light behind it. I was offered an option that would allow me to continue in a role I was good at and to shy away from obsolescence. After much thought and discussion with close friends, I resigned from the clinical arm of my position, maintaining my university faculty professorship. This would allow me several continued teaching options, including teaching medical students on clinical rounds and at the simulation center, doing professor rounds for critical care fellows, and interviewing and assessing applicants to the university medical college. I am frequently invited to write editorials and am still speaking at meetings. I maintain my office and can wander around the hospital ad lib with my starched white coat and physician ID.

For a while, I was somewhat depressed about losing my clinical privileges, but in the end I realized it had to happen someday and it was better to go out on top rather than wait for the inevitable. Having gotten used to the idea, I think my teaching status is a very good gig and I'm very happy and satisfied with it. I've been doing patient care for 30 years and I have a lot to teach. I can maintain this gig pretty much as long as I want to and it's "part-time," so I have more time to work on my bucket list. I'm benefiting my department, and it's gone out of its way to benefit me. My department offered me mutually beneficial options that saved the quality of my life.

Aftermath: The Road Meanders

This intensely personal account of a sudden, unexpected personal illness, my reaction to it, and some very intense thoughts about the nature of aging for otherwise functional physicians concludes here. That said, the issue of aging for direct patient care physicians is still very much an open one, and in my research I found little written about it.

When I was 25, the road ahead of me was very clear. It was only a matter of finding effective and creative ways to stay on that road; I would eventually reach my destination—my dream, if you will. Now, at age 72, I look back. It's much like the end of *Saving Private Ryan* (2012), where the old man, standing in front of Captain Miller's headstone, turns to his family and asks them to reaffirm that he was a good man. It's like Hal Moore, in *We Were Soldiers* (2012), going back to Ia Drang and weeping bitterly over the cost of the path that put him in his present reality.

The reality is that at age 72, the road in front of me no longer leads to the same goal. I have lived the goal beyond my wildest expectations, and now the road has come to an open field, where no matter which way I turn, the scenery changes little. When I proceed, it's into the abstract, and when I turn around, my goals are all behind me and now I contemplate what remains of my future.

For the aging talent, the issue isn't depression; it's facing the possibility of becoming irrelevant. Ernest Hemingway got old and tired and no longer enjoyed his life [4]. David Foster Wallace succumbed to crippling depression, unable to resolve his brilliance with everyday life [5]. However, many with previous careers have continued spectacular successes at ages older than mine. Sir Paul McCartney, Ringo Starr, Eric Clapton, Bob Seger, and the Rolling Stones are still making original music. Doom and gloom isn't inevitable, just looming, waiting to see if it's allowed to be expressed. Aging physicians must find a way to be at peace with growing older and to actively avoid becoming irrelevant. "Some roads you shouldn't go down … 'There be dragons [there]'" [6].

Epilogue: Peace Comes to All… Someday

The reality is that there are more yesterdays in my life than tomorrows, and the yesterdays are fading. My bucket list now looms large. There are a lot of things I want to do and see to round out my life experience. The bucket list is now a live, palpable thing, as much in front of me as the road I faced at age 25.

I have no interest in going gently into that good night. Perhaps I yearn for a *Somewhere in Time*, where Chris Reeves desires to go back so intensely and approximates himself into a time warp so accurately that he actually does return to the past and is given a chance to take another path. But alas, although it might be possible to have it transiently at the end, the coin always lurks that brings it all tumbling down.

And so we come back to the clearing at the end of our road and make what we can of it.

References

1. Derfel A. McGill's medical program put on 'probation' for falling short of standards. Montreal Gazette. June 17, 2015. Available at: http://montrealgazette.com/news/local-news/mcgills-medical-program-put-on-probation-for-falling-short-of-standards.
2. Thompson HS. Fear and loathing: on the campaign trail'72. New York: Simon & Schuster Paperbacks; 2012.
3. Gonzo: The life and work of Dr. Hunter S. Thompson [DVD]. Magnolia Home Entertainment; 2008.
4. Hemingway dead of shotgun wound; wife says he was cleaning weapon. New York Times. July 3, 1961. Available at: https://www.nytimes.com/books/99/07/04/specials/hemingway-obit.html.
5. Weber B. David Foster Wallace, influential writer, dies at 46. New York Times. September 14, 2008. Available at: http://www.nytimes.com/2008/09/15/books/15wallace.html?_r=0.
6. Hawley N. *Fargo*, season 1, episode 1, aired April 15, 2014 (FX).

Chapter 2
The Productive Years: "The Diesel Effect"

Joseph Lex

The editor asked me for "my particular perspective" in becoming an emergency physician/educator/innovator/traveler. First disclaimer: I am an emergency physician – residency trained and board certified – so my perspective may not apply to other critical care specialists. Second disclaimer: I was incredibly lucky, finding opportunities and mentors along the way that I can only wish for others. And third disclaimer: my wife and I decided early in our relationship that we did not want children; this decision made it possible for me to do many things that people raising a family would never be able to do.

After graduating from high school in the suburbs of Chicago in 1965, I set out halfheartedly to study engineering at University of Illinois's Chicago branch. I trudged through the first year of studies without much ambition or success and thought I would take a few months to gather my wits and develop a plan before continuing. But this was, of course, during the Vietnam War and the draft was snapping up young eligible men left and right. Once my student deferment ran out, I became a prime target and was drafted into the US Army in October 1966, initially to serve for 2 years. I realized that with my lack of any skills, my eventual destination was infantry, so I visited a local Army recruitment center to see how I might alter my fate. The recruiting sergeant suggested that I could apply for training as a pharmaceutical tech, but I would have to be a volunteer rather than a draftee to make this happen. So I signed on for an extra year.

After basic training at Fort Campbell, Kentucky, I was assigned to my medical future: combat medic training at Fort Sam Houston in San Antonio, Texas. This 10-week program began in January 1967, and I mark it as the beginning of my career in emergency medicine. I was doing well enough in training that I was offered an opportunity to do further training as a "clinical specialist" – a 40-week program

J. Lex, MD
Department of Emergency Medicine, Temple University Medical Center,
Philadelphia, PA, USA
e-mail: Joseph.Lex@tuhs.temple.edu

© Springer International Publishing Switzerland 2016
D. Crippen (ed.), *The Intensivist's Challenge: Aging and Career Growth
in a High-Stress Medical Specialty*, DOI 10.1007/978-3-319-30454-0_2

offered at a handful of military hospitals around the country. The catch: a full 2-year commitment *after* completing the program. But it was a chance to learn more medicine and – let's face it – delay the inevitable trip to a combat zone. I went to Valley Forge General Hospital in Phoenixville, PA, just 30 miles from Philadelphia. A combination of classroom and bedside teaching gave me the equivalent training of a licensed practical nurse, and I left the school as SP5 E-5, technical equivalent of a sergeant.

The next stop was, of course, Vietnam. Arriving in May 1968, I was assigned to the 1st Battalion, 5th Infantry (Mechanized), 25th Infantry Division with base camps at Cu Chi, Tây Ninh, and Dầu Tiếng. I spent most of my field time at the Battalion Aid Station, dealing with shrapnel wounds, trench foot, and other mostly minor ailments. I also controlled the supply of methylphenidate, which we handed out to soldiers going on night missions. Sometimes I would venture out with a unit on patrol if the company was short in medics, but the majority of my time was in the relative safety of the base camp. Every week or so, we would head to a local village with an interpreter for a MEDCAP – or Medical Civil Action Program – evaluating Vietnamese citizens and their minor injuries or medical problems. To my knowledge, I was the only medic in my unit to *not* receive a Purple Heart for injury in action. I did, however, earn a Combat Medic Badge and a promotion to SP6 (E-6), and our battalion won the Presidential Unit Citation for the Battle of Bến Củi Rubber Plantation [1].

My next assignment was in the orthopedic intake unit at Fort Gordon, in Augusta, Georgia. I reported for duty in June 1969 and spent my last 7 months sorting and caring for young men with some of the most devastating combat injuries you can imagine. Although technically not due for discharge until April 1970, I applied for "early out" in order to try college again at the University of Illinois. I received my honorable discharge in late January 1970 and moved to central Illinois.

I also applied for something new that was being introduced at Duke University: a new category of practitioner called "physician assistant" [2]. At the time, they were taking only navy corpsmen and my application was rejected.

I was not encouraged to pursue medicine at the University of Illinois, where the career counselor told me, "You're nearly 23 years old. By the time you finish your bachelors, you'll be 27 and that's too old for medical school."

From 1970 to 1975 is my "lost years." I was in and out of college a few times, but never stayed long enough to accomplish much. I had a series of dead-end jobs: dishwasher, overnight janitor in a department store, maintenance man in a coal-burning power plant, and deckhand on the Illinois River. One bitterly cold morning as I stood on the head of a barge guiding it into a tow, I realized that there probably was something to getting a higher education. But the next attempt at college – I think it was my fourth – also ended in failure.

From 1972 to 1975, I worked at a small radio station as music director and announcer, and I learned a ton about music. When it became apparent that the station was going to be sold, I started thinking about a new job. One of my radio friends had taken a job as a night registrar at a local hospital emergency department and said they were looking for someone with casting and suturing experience to work the 3–11 shift. "I can do that," I thought, so I eased my way back into medicine as an emergency technician in 1975.

After a few months of working with registered nurses, I thought to myself "I can do that" and decided to investigate a degree in nursing. A local community college offered an associate degree after 2 years of study. I still had enough GI bill left to pay my tuition, and the state of Illinois was paying Vietnam veterans a monthly stipend of $100 to help meet expenses. So while continuing to work full time, I completed a 2-year course in nursing, finishing in 1979 at age 31. I also became school newspaper editor during my second year.

But the hospital where I had worked as a tech for more than 3 years told me they had a policy of not hiring new graduate nurses in the ER. I had no interest in working anywhere else in the hospital, so I searched elsewhere for employment. My girlfriend (now my wife) Andrea, who was a graphic designer, decided her job opportunities were best in either Seattle or Dallas. We drove from Central Illinois to Seattle only to find there was a glut of nurses and they weren't hiring. I drove to Dallas myself and, after interviews at a few hospitals, took a job at Presbyterian Hospital in North Dallas.

Two things happened here to push me forward. First, I had never worked with interns before. When I saw what they did and what they knew, I told myself "I can do that" and started thinking about medical school in earnest. Second, I obtained my first real mentor. Although Compton Broders was about my age, he was a real doctor and I was a nurse. He apparently saw something in me that I had not seen in myself and started pushing. He insisted that I would be a fool if I didn't go to medical school and if I did not I would regret it for the rest of my life. I started taking classes at a local community college – lab courses on Monday through Wednesday and other elective courses on Thursday and Friday mornings. I continued to work at Presbyterian Hospital as a nurse, Thursday and Friday from 3 pm to 11 pm, then Saturday and Sunday from 11 am to 11 pm. It was at this time that my professional nursing organization EDNA (Emergency Department Nurses Association, now simply ENA) developed a certification exam, which I took and passed in July 1980, becoming a member of the first group of nurses to claim the title certified emergency nurse (CEN) [3].

In 2 years I accumulated enough credit hours to apply for medical school. I had done only so-so on the science portions of the MCAT exam but scored very high marks in the reading and comprehension sections. In addition, the philosophy of medical schools had changed, and they were going out of their way to take older students with life experiences. I got interviews at three in-state medical schools and was accepted at University of Texas Health Science Center in San Antonio to begin in 1982. Andrea and I packed and moved to San Antonio. Almost 35 years old, I thought that I would be the "old guy" in the class. It turns out I wasn't even in the top ten.

I was a horrible medical student for the first year. I struggled through with barely a C- average and managed to get to the second year only by the skin of my teeth. For some foolish reason, I had run for class vice president and had been elected. About halfway through the year, the elected president dropped out of medical school – and

I ascended to the presidency. To have a Yankee president in a Texas medical school was almost unheard of, but I apparently met the needs of my 200 classmates because they reelected me three more times and I was still president when I graduated.

When we got out of basic sciences into actually studying medicine, my grades improved significantly. And in the third year, where we finally went to the wards and took care of sick people, I hit my stride. I ended up graduating in the top half of my class – not a superstar by any means but a respectable finish after what had been a ragged start.

As I had been living in Texas since 1979, I was officially a resident and therefore paid in-state tuition. This was during a time when there was an oil glut in the state and tons of money were being shoveled into public education. My tuition for the first 2 years of medical school was … $300/year. The third year it went up to $600 and then it was a whopping $1200 for the fourth year. I worked every other weekend at a nearby community hospital ER from 11 am to 11 pm, earning enough money to keep my debt to a minimum. I borrowed $5000/year and graduated with a debt of only $20,000.

In other words, I attended nursing school on the GI bill and got a free education. Then I attended medical school for next to nothing. This made me a huge proponent of free open access medical education. When I read the Hippocratic Oath, I realized that this may have been the intention of the founder of modern medicine: "To hold him who has taught me this art as equal to my parents and to live my life in partnership with him … and to regard his offspring as equal to my brothers … and to teach them this art—if they desire to learn it—without fee and covenant."

I knew that I only wanted to practice emergency medicine. In fact, I had already determined that if I could not get into an emergency medicine training program, I would continue working as a certified emergency nurse for as long as it took to get into the appropriate training. In 1985 when I applied for a residency, there were fewer than 60 training programs in the country. After spending 7 years in Texas, I let Andrea choose where our next move would be. She handed me back the list: "Chicago, Denver, and Philadelphia." Those were the only cities where I did rotations and the only places where I applied. I did an early rotation at Thomas Jefferson University Hospital in Philadelphia and apparently impressed the powers that be. Although I ranked them third, that is where I found myself going after match day.

Andrea and I quickly adopted Philadelphia as our new home. I learned the skills of emergency medicine over a 3-year training program and made lifelong friends. The Jefferson Emergency Medicine program had been started by pediatrician Joe Zeccardi, and he became my next role model and mentor. I knew that I wanted to go into academics, but felt that I had nothing to offer as a teacher until I had a few years of practice under my belt.

In the days before limited hours of training, I started moonlighting in the emergency department at Germantown Hospital, an inner city community hospital with a lot of "drop off" trauma. It was here I performed my first cricothyrotomy and resuscitative thoracotomy. The patient with the cric survived. In the initial adrenaline rush of doing a thoracotomy, I'd neglected to consider what I would do with the patient after I cross-clamped his aorta. Despite our best efforts he died, saving me the awkward job of transferring a patient with a clamshell chest opening to a nearest trauma center. I made enough money in residency and from moonlighting that I paid off my meager medical school debt and finished the residency debt free. I finished residency training in 1989 and, at age 42, was ready to be an ER doc.

My first job as an attending physician was at Brandywine Hospital and trauma center in Coatesville, PA. It was a single coverage rural hospital with a level II trauma center and a helipad. I would estimate my "ramp up" speed to becoming a competent ER doc was about 2 years. I started giving educational talks, first to the department and then to the hospital staff. Pretty soon I was branching out to local fire stations, Rotary Clubs, and nursing homes. I discovered that I had a knack for delivering a message in such a way that people seemed to understand and learn. I offered myself to the state specialty organization for their annual scientific assembly and gave my first regional talk in 1992.

It was also during this time that I decided I liked working weekends. The hospital was 35 miles from my front door, and weekday traffic was getting insufferable. In 1990 I volunteered to work 12 h shifts on Friday, Saturday, and Sunday. It made my life a lot easier. Since then I have worked almost exclusively weekend shifts. Initially it was days and nights, but I was eventually able to negotiate my way into evening shifts and, excepting backup call-ins, I have not worked a scheduled night shift in more than 20 years.

After 5 years of a long commute, I decided to look at academic positions in Philadelphia. At the time, there were no desirable jobs available, so I took a job at another community hospital, Chestnut Hill Hospital in the northwest corner of the city. I liked the boss, Rick Martin, a lot and we have become fast friends. Again, we are the same age, but he served the role of my next mentor and encouraged me to branch out from the day-to-day practice of emergency medicine. I took the job on a handshake and spent the next 9 years at this community teaching hospital work with family medicine residents, physician assistant and nurse practitioner students, and varying medical students who were rotating through to see if emergency medicine was the specialty for them. In retrospect, I have had several people tell me that they chose emergency medicine as a specialty after working with me and seeing what I was doing and how much fun I was having.

As a firm believer in bedside teaching, I actually went to the bedside when someone wanted to give me the report on a patient. We discussed the entire presentation at bedside in the presence of relatives, allowing for immediate additions and corrections. We discussed the differential diagnosis and if the resident or student didn't mention the word "cancer" or "stroke" or whatever serious condition the patient was probably worried about, then I did it. When we walked away from the bedside, the trainee, the patient, and the family all knew what we were thinking about and what would happen next. I have continued bedside teaching in this manner to this day for any medical student or intern wanting to tell me about a patient. While my colleagues tell me "I don't have time to do that," I found that it actually saved an incredible amount of time. Despite evidence that it improves diagnostic skills and the satisfaction of patients, learners, and teachers, it is a dying art [4].

Despite being at a nonuniversity hospital, I was getting more chances to teach. I had developed a reputation as a good speaker with innovative ideas, and I started getting invited to speak at some local residency training programs, giving the perspective of a community emergency physician with academic aspirations.

The American College of Emergency Physicians (ACEP) had been around for many years; I had joined while I was still a nurse and was given number A24 as an auxiliary member. I continued my membership through my years of training. Even after I became a board certified emergency physician, ACEP allowed me to keep my membership number except, by then, it had to be six digits. Hence, whenever this organization of more than 32,000 emergency medicine specialists generates a list of its members, A000024 always is at the top.

I had heard about a new emergency specialty organization forming. The American Academy of Emergency Medicine (AAEM) was established in 1993 to promote fair and equitable practice environments necessary to allow emergency physicians to deliver the highest quality of patient care. I became a charter member after attending its first Scientific Assembly in Philadelphia in 1994. I heard educational talks that were at a different level than I had heard at other meetings: useful practical information for practicing ER docs, not cut-and-dried information directly from textbooks or journal articles. I have attended every scientific assembly since that first one.

During residency I had developed a talk on wounds suffered by assassinated American presidents, using both medical primary sources and history books. As more people heard the talk, its reputation spread and I received many more invitations to speak. When ACEP had its Scientific Assembly in Philadelphia in 2000, the Pennsylvania Chapter had a welcome reception at the Mütter Museum, a place of wondrous medical curiosities located in the College of Physicians. I knew that this would be my chance to get some national exposure. I got permission to use one of the side rooms to set up a projector and screen and put some promotional posters around the venue. I gave my talk on "Gunshot Wounds in Four Assassinated Presidents" to nearly a hundred people from all over the country at 7 pm; apparently word of mouth got around, and at the 8:30 pm version of the talk, all 150 chairs were full and people were standing along the walls. I now started getting invitations to speak at many state and regional meetings and even an invitation to speak at the 2001 ACEP Scientific Assembly in Chicago. Lesson learned: it's difficult to get a reputation as a good teacher if you aren't at an academic institution. Don't be afraid to self-promote.

I was getting more involved in AAEM, but thought something was missing in the organization. If we were to be taken seriously as leaders in education, we needed to have board review courses. To become board certified in emergency medicine, we must pass both a written test and an oral test. I approached the AAEM board of directors and proposed that I develop these courses and they gave me free rein. I concentrated on the oral board course and wrote 30 cases of hypothetical patients in a hypothetical emergency department. At our first gathering in Florida, I had ten examiners … and 12 candidates. AAEM lost money, but had enough faith in the plan that they allowed me to nurture and develop the course. It has now matured to a twice-yearly session in six cities across the USA, preparing as many as 240 candidates every year to take the oral board examination and become board certified; the pass rate of people who take the course is greater than 98 %.

In the meantime, I had also started speaking at the AAEM Scientific Assemblies with some success. I was still working in the community setting, but could bring that experience to the national level for other emergency physicians practicing away from the Ivory Tower environment. I had some ideas that I wanted to try and asked that the board of directors consider me as possible chair of the Education Committee; I was assigned the job in 2000 and developed the next five national scientific assemblies. It was a brave decision for AAEM to choose a "nonacademic" as chair of its Education Committee. But we were now considered a force to be reckoned with as far as education; despite being only 1/5 the size of ACEP, we had a reputation of giving excellent educational products to our members. Amazingly, we have not charged our members for Scientific Assembly for many years, considering it a member benefit.

Among the ideas I introduced were the open microphone sessions and the Pecha Kucha sessions. Open mic is just an opportunity for someone to show up on the day of the conference and give a 25-min talk on whatever topic they want in front of members of the education committee; in other words, an audition. It had taken me about 10 years to get onto the speaker's circuit, and I hoped this would be a way for others to jump-start their teaching careers. It has been highly successful and even adopted by other organizations. The first year we did it, a young fresh-out-of-residency graduate gave a fantastic talk on "How to Accurately Read a Head CT"; we invited her back the next year to give that talk as part of the formal scientific assembly. Since then, Michelle Lin has gone on to become one of the leaders in emergency medicine education, and her website www.ALiEM.org is a go-to place for current information. Now the open mic is a little more formal and many of the slots are signed up for in advance of the meeting, but true to the "open microphone" philosophy, at least four speaking slots are left open for whoever wants to take advantage of them at the meeting.

Pecha Kucha (PK) is Japanese for chitchat. A PK session is short and to the point: you get to show 20 slides and you spend 20 s on each slide. Six minutes and forty seconds … and done. We took a chance on making this a regular part of our scientific assembly, and it was a major success. It is a win-win-win situation: the audience got seven or eight talks (hence seven or eight take-home points) per hour, the person giving the talk got credit for giving a talk at a national meeting, and AAEM got several hours of strong educational material without paying a dime for the speakers. We have expanded the PK sessions to two full days and even had about 20 of them at a recent international meeting in Rome.

My educational work with AAEM resulted in them naming their "Educator of the Year Award" in 2006; it is now the "Joe Lex Award." A few years later, they honored me again by naming me first recipient of the "Master of American Academy of Emergency Medicine" (MAAEM) award.

In 2001, I was invited to speak at the first Mediterranean Emergency Medicine Conference (MEMC-1) in Stresa, Italy. This was a meeting assembled by AAEM and the European Society of Emergency Medicine. It became a biannual event. I got more involved and became the education chair for versions III and IV and then executive chair for versions V, VI, and VII. Our most recent edition was MEMC-VIII in Rome during 2015, and I gave two talks.

Also in 2001 I was invited to speak at the first EurAsian Emergency Medicine Congress in Istanbul scheduled for the first week of October. After the events of September 11, most of the speakers who had been scheduled to attend dropped out. But the organizers refused to back down and insisted the meeting would take place. I had developed rather significant pulmonary emboli on the flight back from Stresa, Italy, and was taking heparin and warfarin. But I was bound and determined to speak in Istanbul; in order to fill the gaps left by canceling speakers, I gave seven talks. This impressed many international emergency medicine leaders, and I started getting invited to more international meetings.

While international teaching is very rewarding and the idea of bringing my specialty to the rest of the world is quite appealing, it is an expensive hobby; most countries do not have money to fly teachers over the ocean; if we're lucky, they will get us hotel rooms. But their hospitality is always marvelous, with food and drink flowing freely. But if you want to make an impression as an educator in the world at large, be prepared to spend your own money to make it happen. Along the way I have become a charter member of the African Federation for Emergency Medicine and the Vietnamese Society of Emergency Medicine, a full member of the European Society for Emergency Medicine, and an honorary member of Sociedad Argentina de Emergencias (Argentina) and Polskie Towarzystwo Medycyny Ratunkowej (Poland). Because of extensive networking on several continents, I am able to connect people through my personal network. I jokingly say that I am no more than two degrees of separation from everyone in the specialty; I don't know everyone, but I probably know someone who can get in touch with the person you are looking for.

While developing the board review courses for AAEM, I found that I had a knack for writing pretty good board-quality questions: stem worded in a positive manner followed by a correct answer with three or four incorrect distractors. I pored over our major textbooks and came up with 1300 questions covering the breadth of emergency medicine. I gave the book to the Pennsylvania chapter of ACEP and to AAEM to be used by people taking their board review courses. Eventually I published a version with McGraw-Hill, and the questions were incorporated into the question banks of emergency medicine certifying bodies in Poland, Argentina, Iran, Turkey, and Holland.

In 2003, several things happened that made me pursue a new position, this time full time in academics. While I loved the patients and my coworkers at Chestnut Hill Hospital, I was spending more and more time on the road speaking and teaching. My wife was concerned with a large drop in my salary and asked if I could not get a job where this sort of teaching was actually compensated. I interviewed at a few residency training programs in Philadelphia but was most attracted to Temple University – a relatively new residency with a dynamic, ethical, and well-known chair, Robert McNamara. I was hired and immediately placed in charge of resident education and departmental CME. I started bringing outside speakers to teach the residents, and I made available other learning materials by getting department-wide access to such educational programs as Emergency Medical Abstracts and Audio Digest Emergency Medicine. A physician from Massachusetts, Rick Nunez, had contacted me about his new website, www.EMedHome.com, and I started contributing one or two essays annually, along with recordings on our didactic sessions and sending them to be placed on his website. Another acquaintance, Mel Herbert, had decided to start his own continuing medical education program called Emergency Medicine Reviews and Perspectives, so I sent him recordings of our didactic sessions, and he used many of them in the early editions of EMRAP.

After I had accumulated more than 100 recordings, I decided to make them available to whomever wanted them over the Internet. I converted everything to relatively low-fidelity audio at 32 kbps and started posting them on an ftp site, www.YouSendIt.com (now www.hightail.com). I publicized their availability through such LISTSERVs as EMED-L and CCM-L and then watched as they were downloaded initially dozens of times and eventually hundreds of times. This encouraged me to record even more, so I took my trusty recording equipment to regional and state, then international meetings, and recorded and posted more. Eventually one of my residents helped me start a website, www.FreeEmergencyTalks.net, which now has more than 2400 talks available for streaming or download and has been accessed more than a million times. I intentionally made the files as small as possible, so they could be more easily downloaded in countries with limited Internet access.

The website gave me a reputation in the developing world of social media-based education, and I met many more people with similar ideas about the best ways to distribute free education to a motivated group. Dozens of other practitioners and teachers have joined this worldwide movement, and today virtually the entire curriculum of emergency medicine and critical care is available online to any motivated learner to use. This revolutionary movement has caused a seismic shift in the way that young medical students and trainees are educated around the world. Because of my early involvement, I was dubbed "The Godfather of FOAMed."

I moved up the academic ladder successfully, despite doing no research and having only online publications. I had started giving an annual talk on "New Drugs That Might Change Your Practice" in the year 2000 and then was encouraged to write it as an annual article for www.EMedHome.com. I was able to dissect the material in ways that people found it easy to digest and had again found a niche: I was the skeptic who told people what they needed to know about new drugs on the market, most of which provided no benefits over previously available drugs. I then developed other nonclinical talks on "The FDA: Watchdog without a Bite, and with No Incentive to Bark" and "The Drug Shortage: What Happened?" This led to invitations to speak at hospital grand rounds and even law schools. Because of my national, and then international, reputation as an educator in emergency medicine, I was promoted at Temple University from assistant professor to associate professor to clinical professor in the minimum required time – 5 years at each level. I reached full professorship in 2013, 10 years after taking my first academic job and shortly before moving to part-time status. Lesson learned: the traditional "publish or perish" may no longer be a valid path to academic legitimacy. Enlightened academic institutions are seeing the value of their faculty becoming involved in newer, nontraditional methods of teaching: blogs, podcasts, and even Twitter.

I have been quoted as saying, "If you want to know how we are going to practice emergency medicine in the future, listen to the conversations in the hallway and use FOAMed." Blogs, podcasts, Google® hangouts, text documents, photographs, web-based applications, etc., are the lifeblood of FOAMed. There are more than 240 bloggers and podcasters putting out material on almost a daily basis. And Twitter is a world in itself, with conversations sprouting over controversial topics within minutes and continuing for days. A landmark article is discussed on the same day as publication. A new technique is disseminated around the world within hours: a good example is the recent series of tweets concerning bougie-guided thoracostomy tube placement. Links to free articles, videos, and blogs appear at a dizzying rate if you follow the right Tweeters.

I retire from clinical medicine at the end of June 2016, perhaps by the time you read this, after 491/2 years in emergency medicine. I leave the future of emergency medical education in the hands of people like Haney Mallemat (@CriticalCareNow), Anand Swaminathan (@EMSwami), Scott Weingart (@EMcrit), Michelle Lin (@M_Lin), and Rob Rogers (@EM_Educator), among dozens of others. They too are passionate about FOAM and will be on the frontlines for the next 20 or 30 years. The change to FOAM will not take place overnight, but it will take place. As Max Planck wisely noted, "A new scientific truth does not triumph by convincing its opponents and making them see the light, but rather because its opponents eventually die, and a new generation grows up that is familiar with it" [5]. The future is inevitable: FOAMed will replace textbooks and journals. Lead, follow, or get out of the way. And don't make your age an excuse: in my third year of receiving Social Security checks, I have nearly 6000 followers on Twitter.

I will be nearly 69 years old and despite a rigorous exercise program and biannual hikes of 90+ miles, I feel age tugging at my sleeve. I lose simple words that I have used for decades. I struggle to understand new concepts such as rotational thromboelastometry (ROTEM) and extracorporeal membrane oxygenation (ECMO). I have lost many procedural skills by virtue of practicing in a teaching environment, where preference must be given to the learner. In my 13 years in academia, I have done two orotracheal intubations, two nasotracheal intubations, and two cricothyrotomies. My trainees are that good. They run circles around me with their ultrasound skills. I do not want to get to the stage where people say, "He used to be a good ER doc." A good friend retired last year, saying "I prefer to retire 2 or 3 years too early rather than 10 minutes too late." I will continue to teach, if people will have me, but it will not be clinical emergency medicine. I can usually spot a nonclinician less than 5 min into a talk – the passion about medicine and patient care just isn't there.

My next career will be with young jazz musicians. Mentoring young intelligent, motivated people is the same no matter what the field. And in emergency medicine, just as in jazz, we tend to make it up as we go along. But it's been an amazing journey in emergency medicine. Next to Ringo Starr, I consider myself the luckiest man on the planet.

References

1. 5th Infantry Regiment Association. Ben Cui August 21, 1968. http://www.bobcat.ws/ben-cui-tribute.html.
2. Physician Assistant History Society. 1957 to 1970: The Formative Years. http://www.pahx.org/period02.html.
3. Board of Certification for Emergency Nursing. BCEM History. https://www.bcencertifications.org/About-BCEN/History.aspx.
4. Peters M, Ten Cate O. Bedside teaching in medical education: a literature review. Perspect Med Educ. 2014;3(2):76–88.
5. Wissenschaftliche Selbstbiographie. Mit einem Bildnis und der von Max von Laue gehaltenen Traueransprache. Johann Ambrosius Barth Verlag (Leipzig 1948), p. 22, as translated in Scientific Autobiography and Other Papers, trans. F. Gaynor (New York, 1949), pp. 33–34 (as cited in T. S. Kuhn, The Structure of Scientific Revolutions).

Chapter 3
The Aging Intensivist and Business Management

John W. Hoyt

Introduction

It was the academic year 1971/1972 and I was a straight Medicine intern at the Good Samaritan Hospital in Cincinnati. I had graduated from the University of Cincinnati College of Medicine and had cardiology in the back of my mind for fellowship training. Fourteen members of the UC class of 106 went to Good Samaritan because of its strong teaching program in Medicine. There were ICU rotations in a 16-bed intensive care unit and patients intubated on pressure-limited ventilators. We had arterial lines connected to mercury columns and Swan-Ganz catheters connected to water columns. Unfortunately, we had no idea what we were doing in the ICU and little to no supervision of our diagnostic and therapeutic plans. The hospital had an open heart surgery program which provided expertise from anesthesia, cardiology, and cardiac surgery. The specialty of Critical Care was in the birthing process, and we all did the best we could to learn and provide good care. By the end of the year, I had a sense I wanted to work in the ICU but assumed that would happen through cardiology.

By the spring of 1972, my military obligation related to Vietnam was coming due. I had signed up for the senior medical student program and spent a year collecting an ensign's salary with the US Navy. My wife was a teacher in the Cincinnati public schools and money was in short supply. I knew by the middle of medical school that I would be drafted to serve because of the Barry Plan. I made a decision to get paid as a senior student and help with the debt. As I approached the completion of my internship and the time to begin my active duty,

J.W. Hoyt, MD, MCCM
Pittsburgh Critical Care Associates, Inc., Pittsburgh, PA, USA

Clinical Professor of Critical Care Medicine, University of Pittsburgh Medical Center, Pittsburgh, PA, USA
e-mail: HoytJ@pccaintensivist.com

© Springer International Publishing Switzerland 2016
D. Crippen (ed.), *The Intensivist's Challenge: Aging and Career Growth in a High-Stress Medical Specialty*, DOI 10.1007/978-3-319-30454-0_3

an unexpected event changed my life and initiated a career in critical care. I got a letter from the Navy asking if I wanted 6 free months of anesthesia training (free means no payback time). Because of my experience with anesthesia at Good Samaritan, and the obvious ICU expertise of the cardiac anesthesiologists, it seemed appropriate to accept the offer of free training in procedures such as intubation, ventilation, and resuscitation. Somewhere in the back of my mind, I had to know that meant a trip to front lines in Vietnam. Looking back with more mature eyes, a trip to Vietnam when we already had one child may not have been the best idea.

By the spring of 1972, I got a letter from the US Navy asking me to pick in order of preference which Naval Hospital I wanted for my anesthesia support training. I listed Philadelphia, Boston, and Great Lakes. They sent me to Naval Regional Medical Center Portsmouth, Virginia, which was not on the list. I showed up for active duty in July after being promoted to Lieutenant. I met the Chief of Anesthesia, Dr. William McDermott. He informed me that he had registered me with the American Board of Anesthesia as a first year resident. Dr. McDermott explained that this was a first year class of anesthesia residents for Portsmouth. NRMC Portsmouth was a 1200-bed hospital with most of the key residencies but not anesthesia. Somewhere a decision was made by the Navy to start a new residency. Dr. McDermott told me that if I did not like doing anesthesia, he could find some place to put me. After two weeks of grumbling, I finally acquiesced to the will of the US Navy and reframed myself as an anesthesiologist with a very strong interest in critical care. In the negotiations, Dr. McDermott told me he would find a critical care fellowship for me when my anesthesia training was completed.

By the spring of 1974, Dr. McDermott had been reassigned from Portsmouth to Washington and was in the Bureau of Personnel. In a phone conversation with Dr. McDermott, he confirmed the deal we had made and told me to look at critical care fellowships. We agreed the Navy would pay for the training.

The Barry Plan, or doctor draft as it was known, served military residents in training very well. There were 12 Barry Plan anesthesia faculty at Portsmouth. They were from the best anesthesia training programs in the country including Pittsburgh, Boston, and Philadelphia. One anesthesia Pittsburgh faculty member in Portsmouth, Bob Binda, M.D., was trained in pediatric critical care and strongly recommended the University of Pittsburgh Critical Care fellowship that had been started by Peter Safar, M.D., and Ake Grenvik, M.D. Another anesthesia faculty member in Portsmouth, Ron Brons, M.D., had trained at the Massachusetts General Hospital and worked in the ICU with Henning Pontoppidan, M.D. I visited both programs and chose Pittsburgh. To this day, it is not clear that one program was better than the other. They were both very young training programs and reflected the youthful nature of this new specialty. When I arrived in Pittsburgh, there were 14 fellows. UPMC gave me all the science behind the things I had seen in the ICU at Good Samaritan in Cincinnati. Having said that, I will never understand how these series of improbable events involving the US Navy and Vietnam provided me with such a satisfying career in the practice of medicine.

Clinical Manager

This chapter is dedicated to "the aging intensivist as manager." Most people would look at my past history over the last 40 years and say that I was a clinician and manager. When it comes to the practice of medicine and especially critical care, there are many definitions of a manager. I covered most of those definitions. After finishing my training in July of 1975, I spent 1 year doing anesthesia, pain clinic, and studying for my boards. In July of 1976, I took over as Medical Director of the Medical/Surgical ICU at the Portsmouth Naval Hospital. For a number of years, the Department of Anesthesiology at Portsmouth had managed the ICU. Since I had just gotten back from my CCM fellowship in Pittsburgh, I was an obvious choice to be ICU Director. In fact, the Navy frequently used anesthesiology to manage hospital intensive care units as they did at Bethesda Naval Hospital in Washington where Myer Rosenthal, M.D., was ICU Director. Little did I know the issues I would face. From my training, I was used to an all registered nurse staff with a ratio of one nurse for two patients. That was not the Navy way. The Navy used one corpsman per patient with 6 patients and 6 corpsman supervised by one nurse. The corpsman had been trained for general duty and not for the intensive care unit. As the manager of the unit, I embarked on ICU training for the corpsman and the nurses.

The existing monitoring equipment in the ICU was from the early1960s – functional but not useful for general duty corpsman. The Navy allowed me to purchase all new monitors so that I had the ability to measure pressure for arterial, central, and pulmonary artery lines at each bedside. We had a central station and even a computer to store lab work. I kept census information so that I could supply the admiral with monthly reports to justify my need for more corpsman and nurses.

This was a busy ICU with lots of sick patients and a great opportunity for residents to learn about managing patients with life-threatening illnesses. By meeting with the Chief of Medicine and Chief of Surgery, I was able to create ICU rotations for residents from surgery, medicine, and anesthesiology. There was great support from the medical staff and administration. In that setting of ICU management, I was creating a vision learned at the University of Pittsburgh and rolling out that vision at Portsmouth Naval Hospital.

Unfortunately by 1978, Portsmouth was used as a destination for prisoners of war since Vietnam was over. The military was not popular with the country, and the Defense Department budget for healthcare had shrinking dollars. It would take 20 years for the country's attitude to the military to change. I was 33 years old with a wife and three children and it was time to move on. The Navy had been very good to me and set me on a path as a manager of critical care services. It would be hard to underestimate all that I had learned. This learning was not just clinical information but management information about running an ICU, surviving hospital politics, and building alliances and power bases. Ake Grenvik in Pittsburgh had been enormously helpful with that learning. He told all the 1974 fellows to do everything we could to help the hospital so that we were cemented in the fabric of the ICU and people would look at us and judge that they could not live without the services of the critical care manager.

When I started to look for a job, I got offers from the University of Virginia and Wake Forest University. I picked the University of Virginia and started as ICU Director of the Medical/Surgical ICU in July of 1978. Bob Epstein, M.D., was Chairman of the Department of Anesthesiology, and I became an assistant professor in his department. I had been promised a remodeled ICU and a computerized patient data management system. There were three other anesthesiology faculty with critical care training/experience that shared coverage of the ICU. We developed rotations for surgery and anesthesiology residents. I used the same management vision that I had in the Navy. Unfortunately, the University of Virginia was much less willing to change and I was young and brash and determined. Because of a very strong alliance with nursing, we were able to remodel the ICU and install the computer system. We initiated the computerized record for all surgical services except cardiac surgery. They refused to participate.

In 1983, I left the University of Virginia and moved to Pittsburgh. For the last 20 years, I have thought about my 5 years in Charlottesville. I have thought about my youthful and brash style. I have thought about Bob Epstein's best efforts to make it work for me. I have thought about management styles and what it takes to bring an intensivist system to a hospital that has never seen that model of care. Today, across the country, hospitals large and small want to have intensivist programs. Most times they fail to understand what the desire for an intensivist program means. It requires a clear vision, a true desire for change despite all adversity, and a willingness to steel yourself against repeated political attacks attempting to prevent change. Based on 40 years of experience, and hundreds of observations, I believe it is not possible to achieve an intensivist system that improves the quality of care and reduces the cost of care without making huge changes from the time the program starts. I have never seen starting slow and small work to produce a quality product.

Other specialties have endured the same resistance to change. Emergency medicine experienced the same challenges in the 1970s. It took 10–15 years for the value of emergency medicine to be recognized and have emergency departments staffed by residency trained emergency medicine physicians. Anesthesiology has been recognized as an essential hospital-based specialty for decades. There is much less resistance to change. Critical care started with fellowship programs in the late 1960s. It spread slowly and in various formats in academic hospitals. It has been slow to spread to private hospitals. In those private hospitals, pulmonologists do critical care consults, but they don't provide the 24-h in-house coverage that is part of emergency medicine, anesthesiology, and intensivist-based critical care. Over the next 15 years, intensivists will spread to 90 % of moderate- to large-size hospitals dramatically improving the quality of care and saving lives. For that to happen, there has to be a clear vision of an intensivist service and a willingness to make the changes that will allow this revolution to happen. Most importantly, there has to be a cadre of intensivists with skills at management to create these intensivist programs.

I moved to Pittsburgh in 1983 for a position in a private practice Department of Anesthesiology where I was to do operating room anesthesia and run the 18-bed medical/surgical ICU. St. Francis Medical Center was a 750-bed hospital where the medical staff had decided they wanted intensivists in the ICU (quite progressive for 1983). After an extensive interview process and two separate visits, I decided that I could make my acquired vision of the intensivist model work at St. Francis. My anesthesia colleagues were to cover the ICU at night. St. Francis had a big and successful internal medicine residency. These residents covered the ICU at night with supervision by anesthesia. Sister Sylvia Schuler and Sister Rosita Wellinger were the administrative managers of the hospital. In fact, it was Sister Sylvia who, after I turned the job down the first time, called me on the phone in the ICU at the University of Virginia and told me "God wants you at St. Francis Hospital." That was a level of management that was hard to ignore and way exceeded the power and influence of the admiral at the Naval Hospital.

The partnership with the Anesthesia Department at St. Francis was difficult from the beginning. The vision of the covering anesthesiologist for the ICU was putting in endotracheal tubes and arterial lines when the residents needed help. They were not interested in doing medical management of the patients. The hospital was very happy with the daytime intensivist services, but the Department of Anesthesiology wanted out by June of 1989. I had a secure place on the medical staff and with hospital administration and a clinical appointment in Critical Care at the University of Pittsburgh. Critical care fellows from the University of Pittsburgh had started to rotate at St. Francis. At this point, I entered an entirely new form of critical care management. I resigned from my anesthesia role and contracted with the hospital for critical care services.

Business Manager

Up to this point in my intensivist career, I had been a salaried employee with the US Navy, University of Virginia, or the St. Francis Anesthesia Department. Now I was on my own and entered into an entirely new phase of intensivist management. I had to sign a contract with the hospital, create a corporation, develop a billing and collection system, prepare a budget, hire intensivists, and pay salaries and benefits. My mentor through all of this was Elmer Holzinger, M.D., Chief of Medicine and de facto hospital medical director. I sought out a healthcare attorney and a healthcare accounting group and became the business manager of Pittsburgh Critical Care Associates, Inc., an "S" Corporation in the State of Pennsylvania. I would just say that we were quite prosperous and I hired graduating critical care fellows from the UPMC program. We got to 7 intensivists and developed a coverage system with two intensivists on days and one intensivist on nights. Round-the-clock coverage made a big difference in the quality and safety of care. Our reputation in the community grew, and we enlarged the business in the ICU from 4,000 to over 6,000 patient days per year. We developed a transport system to bring patients to St. Francis from outside hospitals. We developed a risk-adjusted database that demonstrated ICU death rate and ICU length of stay was below predicted. My duties and responsibilities were manager of clinical services and manager of business services. This last part I made up on my own as I went along with a good lawyer and a good accountant. Having said that, any intensivist who organizes a group of hospital-based intensivists has to learn to be both a clinical manager and a business manager. Critical Care fellows do not learn this in most CCM fellowship programs. UPMC has created a management course for CCM fellows, and I have been quite privileged to be part of that. CCM fellows leave the fellowship in Pittsburgh with a much better understanding of the business of critical care. It is essential for an ICU manager to understand the process of making money to pay the bills. The Sisters at St. Francis use to say "no margin no mission." Making money should not be reviled as an evil endeavor. Making money drives the business so that intensivists can provide the patient care to save lives. Making money to line the manager's pocket is an evil endeavor and sacrifices patient outcomes.

For 13 years, St. Francis was an ideal intensivist work environment. We were so successful from a management standpoint that the hospital asked us to take over the operation of the four emergency departments in the system. We designed and built a 32-bed intensive care unit that incorporated the coronary care unit. Unfortunately, there were certain administrative issues that we could not monitor. We did not know the cost of care in the ICU. We did not know what the hospital charged for a day in the ICU. We did not know what the hospital got paid for a day in the ICU and what sort of contracts existed with various payers. To this day, I do not know these hospital numbers for any of the 5 intensive care units that we manage. Hospitals rarely understand the cost of care in the ICU and operate on charges rather than revenue and expenses. At St. Francis, that led to financial crises. The hospital completed an aggressive building program but did not have the money to service the debt. That led to the closure of the Medical Center and the three satellite hospitals. Pittsburgh Critical Care had to rapidly downsize its staff at all levels and attempt to survive on several outside contracts. This was clearly a lesson that I needed to learn. Intensivists must understand the "margin" or profit of a hospital. This is profit on operations and not on savings. There are things like cash on hand and savings that are essential to understanding the economic health of the hospital.

Consultant Manager

In trying to rebuild the business base of Pittsburgh Critical Care, we began to get consults from hospitals around the country asking for help in starting intensivist programs. These hospitals were not interested in subcontracting intensivist services but instead learning how to manage an intensivist program with the assistance of an intensivist manager. Using the management experience of the past 26 years, I was able to become successful in starting new programs and demonstrating the effectiveness of these new programs. The eagerness of hospitals to trade out the pulmonary consultation model for the dedicated intensivist model convinces me we are on the edge of a huge growth in intensivist services. In a recent visit to Dublin,

Ireland, I had the opportunity to round with an intensivist in one of the intensive care units. They have used the intensivist model for 30 years. The quality of care is extraordinary and the outcomes are superb. Hopefully, the United States will see similar increases in quality and decreases in cost as the intensivist model spreads across the country.

One of the essential parts of an intensivist business is a strong and loyal infrastructure. The manager must have talented people to manage the financial books, collect outcome data, do billing and collections, recruit good physician intensivists, develop physician schedules and manage the calendar, and monitor physician performance. I have been fortunate to acquire and maintain this infrastructure with people who have been with me for over 25 years. An infrastructure like that is expensive but essential to the success of the clinical and business intensivist program.

Bibliography

1. Wernerman J. The role of the intensive care unit in the modern hospital. In: Flaatten HM, Moreno RP, Putensen C, Rhodes A, editors. Organisation and management of intensive care. Berlin: Medizinisch Wissenschaftliche Verlagsgesellschaft (MWV); 2010. p. 21–6.
2. Streat S. Evaluating and improving the effectiveness of our practices. In: Flaatten HM, Moreno RP, Putensen C, Rhodes A, editors. Organisation and management of intensive care. Berlin: Medizinisch Wissenschaftliche Verlagsgesellschaft (MWV); 2010. p. 295–306.
3. Brilli RJ, Spevetz A, Branson RD, et al. Critical care delivery in the intensive care unit: defining clinical roles and the best practice model. Crit Care Med. 2001;29(10):2007–19.

Chapter 4
The Aging Critical Care Physician: A 50-Year Progression of Events

Ake Grenvik

Lessons Learned During My Career in Critical Care Medicine

This chapter illustrates how thorough postgraduate training and successful research with excellent mentoring directed a young academician into a new and rapidly growing field in high demand and offered the opportunity for a leading position with international reputation and suitable continued involvement into retirement.

Sweden

A native of Sweden I graduated in 1956 from medical school at the Karolinska Institute in Stockholm. I obtained training in anesthesiology and general and cardiothoracic surgery at the Universities of Lund and Uppsala. That included 3 years of clinical research in Uppsala. At the end of their operative procedures, our open heart surgical patients were equipped with right atrium, pulmonary artery, left atrium, and systemic artery catheters. Pressure recording, various blood gas analyses, and cardio-green determination of cardiac output were done. Pulmonary function was studied using pneumotachography providing tracheal pressure and airflow with display of tidal volume and minute ventilation. Intrathoracic pressure was recorded through the chest tubes and oxygen consumption calculated using the Fick principle. Twenty-two cardiac surgical patients were studied postoperatively in the ICU on and off mechanical ventilation.

The results demonstrated how respiratory, circulatory, and metabolic variables changed during mechanical ventilation compared to spontaneous breathing. Current

A. Grenvik, MD, PhD, MCCM
Department of Critical Care Medicine, University of Pittsburgh Medical Center, Pittsburgh, PA, USA
e-mail: grenvik@verizon.net

© Springer International Publishing Switzerland 2016   29
D. Crippen (ed.), *The Intensivist's Challenge: Aging and Career Growth in a High-Stress Medical Specialty*, DOI 10.1007/978-3-319-30454-0_4

opinion that central venous pressure increases with intermittent positive pressure ventilation while cardiac output decreases did not make sense. However, I used differential pressure transducers and measured transmural pressures of the heart and intrathoracic great vessels. Indeed those pressures, including transmural central venous pressure, then decreased during positive-pressure ventilation as cardiac output fell. The physiologic problem was solved. The findings also contributed to earlier weaning from mechanical ventilation and tracheal extubation of our ICU patients. The medical thesis was published in 1966 [1] and resulted in a magna cum laude PhD.

Discussing the usefulness of the scientific publication with my mentors, Viking Bjork, chief of cardiothoracic surgery, and Martin Holmdahl, chief of anesthesiology and later Chancellor of the University, I was advised to consider my future career in anesthesiology and intensive care rather than cardiothoracic surgery. In Scandinavia as well as in many other countries, especially in Europe, anesthesiologists were taking the leadership in intensive care. My thesis was published as a supplement to the Scandinavian anesthesiology journal.

My wife, Inger, was absolutely essential to the entire research. She was my clinical assistant, technician, secretary, and statistician, manually calculating the necessary data as computers were not yet in use. I dictated on a tape recorder and she transcribed the text. As I was running out of funding in the 3rd year, we tried to finish the thesis before the end of that academic year and worked almost around the clock. The book was printed in Denmark, 600 miles from our home in Uppsala. The university required a minimum of 500 books for graduation. Inger and I had to drive down to Denmark and pick up those books ourselves in order to meet the deadline. But on the very last day of this academic year, i.e., May 31, 1966, I was indeed ready for graduation.

Traveling in 1967

The above exhausting finish took its toll. Severely sleep deprived, I still needed to return to clinical work as we were heavily in debt from borrowing money during the 3 years of research. With a family of six, I had not yet paid off my loans from medical school to begin with. When I noticed how my fellow residents had advanced in surgical skills with I myself far behind, I became deeply depressed to the point of developing suicidal thoughts. By chance at this time, I received an invitation to serve as ship's surgeon on the new M/S Kungsholm, preparing for a 3-month cruise around the Pacific Ocean starting in New York City. Both my mother and Inger urged me to accept, which I fortunately did, obtaining a leave of absence from the university. Being professionally busy on the ship and serving as host at one of the tables in the dining theater was excellent treatment of my depression. Already after a week on board, I was feeling much better and life enthusiasm returned to normal.

When the Kungsholm returned to New York City, I left by previous agreement and had the opportunity to travel throughout North America, visiting famous cardiac surgical departments and intensive care units both in the USA and Canada. At the end of my trip, while at the Mayo Clinic, I was called upon by Peter Safar in Pittsburgh. He invited me to lecture on my research findings at his first international emergency and critical care medicine congress. My presentation was well received and I was invited back to Pittsburgh for further training in critical care. Indeed the Safar training program in CCM was the only well-established such program so I happily accepted the invitation.

Pittsburgh

In May 1968, I started as a Pittsburgh fellow in CCM and my family moved over in July. We rented a house when I served as a trainee in the 16-bed general ICU at the Presbyterian University Hospital. We were four fellows that year. The others were one anesthesiologist from Israel (Polly Lieberman), one internist from Switzerland (Claude Bernheim), an internist/pulmonary medicine specialist from South Africa (Jan Smith), and myself mostly trained in surgery but also in anesthesiology. This was the fifth CCM training year in Peter Safar's program, but in the preceding academic years, the trainees were mainly anesthesiology residents. However, now we had different primary specialties represented among the trainees. We agreed that training in CCM should be available to any physician specialist with particular interest in ICU patient problems.

After I completed my fellowship year in CCM, I was asked to take responsibility for directing all aspects of the ICU administration, including patient care, organization, and teaching. Peter Safar left for a sabbatical year of research. At the end of this year, I was offered and accepted a faculty position in the Division of CCM within the Department of Anesthesiology. This was a most attractive offer compared to what I had in Sweden, so I resigned from the University of Uppsala and started my first Pittsburgh faculty position on July 1, 1970. Because of my thorough training in Sweden and the USA, my first appointment was as an associate professor in anesthesiology/CCM. After passing the ABA exam, I was also certified in CCM when this subspecialty exam became available.

Upon their graduation from our program, two outstanding trainees were hired as CCM faculty members. They were James Snyder, an anesthesiologist, and David Powner, an internist. So we had the combination of an anesthesiologist, an internist and a surgeon in the local CCM leadership. These two colleagues became my closest collaborators over many years. Together, we developed a well-working patient care and teaching program. One of the CCM fellows was on call every night. That fellow was familiar with all ICU patients and ready for immediate intervention in case of an emergency. He or she also responded to hospital wide codes to participate in lifesaving measures wherever indicated. I came in early, at 4 am every day, to check on the patients. Together with the fellow on call, I made sure that all patients were stabilized and extubations were performed as indicated in preparation for 7 am rounds, thus not interrupted by foreseeable patient needs. The ICU head nurse participated in these rounds and each bedside nurse as well when his or her patient was discussed while we together agreed on an individual care plan for the day. At 12 noon every day, we had a lecture on a relevant topic. Each Wednesday this was the weekly grand rounds, often with an invited speaker. At about 5 pm we went on evening rounds, summarizing pertinent information and developed a care plan for the upcoming night.

In 1969 Peter Safar appointed Stephan Kampschulte, a German anesthesiologist, as director of the new pediatric ICU at Children's Hospital (CHP). He started a separate pediatric CCM fellowship. Initially we rotated our "adult" CCM fellows through this pediatric ICU and the pediatric CCM fellows had a corresponding rotation through our "adult" ICU. But this had such disadvantages that the arrangement was discontinued and the pediatric CCM fellowship split off as a separate training program in CCM. After a few years, Stephan Kampschulte returned to Germany. Later on, Peter Winter as the current Anesthesiology Chairman recruited Ann Thompson to direct the pediatric CCM program. She was thoroughly trained in two primary specialties, anesthesiology and pediatrics, including CCM at the Hospital for Sick Children in Philadelphia. She became certified by both ABA and ABP in CCM. ABP is the only American board that requires 3 years of CCM training which must include at least 1 year of research. As a consequence, research flourished in the pediatric CCM program at CHP.

CCM Societies

In late 1969 Peter Safar and I went to Los Angeles for the first meeting of a group of 28 intensive care active physicians of various specialties. We agreed that it was time to start a society of critical care medicine (SCCM). Max Harry Weil, internist/cardiologist in Los Angeles, served as our host and was elected as the founding president of SCCM. This society was not limited to a specific primary specialty but rather open to any primary specialty physician whose special interest and activity was in CCM. Indeed the 28 of us founding members represented a wide variety of primary medical specialties, including pediatrics and even neonatology. Possibilities were also developed for nonphysicians, such as ICU nurses, researchers, respiratory therapists, and various technicians in CCM [2] to join the SCCM.

During the second SCCM year, a decision was reached to start a special monthly journal in CCM. Peter Safar was then the SCCM president and appointed William Shoemaker as chief editor. From the onset, he worked tirelessly on the CCM journal and served as the third SCCM president. Again, we had an indication of CCM multidisciplinarity with the first three presidents being an internist, anesthesiologist, and surgeon in that order. Annual SCCM meetings were arranged, initially alternating in a piggyback fashion at the well-functioning annual CCM meetings in Los Angeles and Pittsburgh.

I served as president of SCCM in 1977. During that year work was initiated to establish a multidisciplinary subspecialty board certification in CCM. However, this proved difficult to accomplish. The four American Boards of Anesthesiology, Internal Medicine, Pediatrics, and Surgery together with SCCM formed a committee reporting to the American Board of Medical Specialties. After 2 years of deliberations, the four boards, ABA, ABIM, ABP, and ABS, decided to establish separate subspecialties in CCM. In the mid-1980s, these were approved by the ABMS [3, 4].

Alan Gilston, a renowned cardiac anesthesiologist in the UK, and Iain McA Ledingham, a well-known surgeon directing intensive care at the Royal Infirmary in Glasgow, together arranged the first International Congress on Intensive Care in London in 1974. A few of us invited speakers decided to form a World Federation of Societies of Intensive and Critical Care Medicine (WFSICCM). A constitution advisory committee was appointed with representatives from the UK, France, Switzerland, Scandinavia, Israel, Japan, Australia/New Zealand, Mexico, Canada, and the USA. The proposed constitution was approved at the Second World Congress, taking place in Paris in 1977. It was decided for WFSICCM to meet every 4 years. Alberto Villazon, surgeon/intensivist in Mexico City, was elected first president and I served as treasurer/secretary.

The third WFSICCM congress was held in Washington DC in 1981, combined with the annual SCCM meeting. I was appointed to serve as the program committee chairman. This congress took place at the Washington Hilton Hotel, where President Reagan was shot the preceding year. Because of President Reagan's dramatic hospitalization and successful emergency thoracotomy, all representing well-functioning critical care, we invited him to open our congress. Unfortunately, he had to decline but sent a most appreciated, congratulatory letter to SCCM, which Joe Civetta as the current SCCM president read aloud during the opening ceremony. This SCCM congress was the largest to date but also the most costly.

Fund Raising

I was asked by our current Anesthesia Department chairman, Leonard Firestone, to chair a committee, tasked with the establishment of a Peter Winter-endowed chair in anesthesiology. Having served for 25 years on the Norwegian Board for Acute Medicine at the Laerdal Medical Corporation in Stavanger, I contacted its president, Tore Laerdal since Laerdal Medical had been our by far greatest benefactor over the past decades. Safar's International Resuscitation Research Center and our Division of CCM had received very large grants. But this time, I was informed that it was not in the current interest of the corporation to establish a chair in anesthesiology. Instead I was recommended to apply for a grant to build a simulation center. I had discussed repeatedly with Tore Laerdal the need and possibility for the corporation to construct a human CCM simulator based on their extensive experience and success with Resusci Anne, the CPR training mannequin used all over the world. Peter Winter had the foresight to obtain a human simulator when these were new in the growing field of using simulators in medical education. From the Laerdal

Foundation for Acute Medicine, we obtained a $ 1 M grant and could build a world-class simulation center, which we named WISER standing for the Peter M Winter Institute for Simulation, Education, and Research. My job as chairman of the committee to establish a chair in Peter Winter's name was completed. But instead of a chair, we created an institute in his honor.

Introducing a new medical specialty, over the years, I authored or coauthored some 400 publications on CCM-related topics, varying from physiologic and outcome studies as well as organizational questions in the ICU to transplantation issues, ethical dilemmas, physician training in CCM, and use of simulators in medical education. My publications included 27 books, foremost my medical thesis in 1966 and several editions of the leading Textbook of Critical Care of which I served as chief editor of the 4th edition, published in the year 2000 [5].

Rapid Response Systems

All hospitals had a cardiac arrest code, calling on a team for immediate action in these emergencies. But the results were not good. It occurred to me that most cardiac arrest situations were preceded by symptoms of patient deterioration and during this time it should be possible to treat the patient and often avoid the arrest. At our hospital, we had a Condition A for cardiac arrest. I recommended introduction of the code Condition C standing for crisis and the nurses should have the right to call Condition C whenever the patient's condition turned worrisome. But this was defeated by the ICU committee, since the current American teaching system was to let the intern attack the problem first and call on the resident of the case, if not successful. The resident in turn could then call on the attending physician. But all this took time and the deteriorating patient might then develop cardiac arrest. The golden opportunity to prevent cardiac arrest was lost due to a clumsy system.

I tried for over 1 year to change this. Then something happened. The wife of our surgical department chairman suffered from breast cancer with a suspicious lung metastasis. The oncologist did a transthoracic needle biopsy following which the patient began to deteriorate with dyspnea and falling blood pressure. I was called upon and in turn alerted a CCM fellow, an ICU nurse, and a respiratory therapist, who brought our crash cart. We provided oxygen, started an IV infusion, obtained a chest X-ray, and found a large pneumothorax with fluid in the pleural cavity. We inserted a chest tube which drained air and blood. The patient was transported to the ICU, where her condition improved. In other words, she was treated the way I had outlined in the ICU committee for more than 1 year. At the next ICU committee meeting, the Condition C system was approved without any further problems. In the following years the number of Condition C cases increased and the number of Condition A cases decreased as mortality dropped. Our current CCM faculty member, MichaeL de Vita, picked up on the idea. He arranged international meetings and published a book on this system using what was called rapid response teams, with hospitals all over the world introducing rapid response condition codes.

I traveled frequently and was invited as a speaker at various CCM meetings, nationally and abroad, presenting over 700 lectures in more than 30 countries. My heavy worldwide involvement In CCM contributed greatly to the growth and popularity of our program. During my 20 years of CCM leadership at the University of Pittsburgh, we trained over 500 intensivists. Many of them came from abroad. Upon graduation, they could return home and many became leaders in CCM, locally or regionally. Thus we have satellite CCM programs all over the world.

Family Problem

Life treated me extremely well, until 1987 when disaster struck in our family. Our son Christer graduated from medical school at the University of Miami that year with an unfortunate diagnosis of an incurable glioblastoma multiforme. He died as an anesthesiology resident 2 years later. We parents were devastated and needed to get away from Pittsburgh. I applied for a sabbatical leave and accepted an invitation to work for half a year as a visiting professor at the University of South Florida in Tampa. During this time, Inger and I recovered slowly from our terrible loss and could return back to Pittsburgh. Jim Snyder, who served as interim chief of our CCM Division, did very well, continuing the established tradition in Pitt CCM. Upon return to Pittsburgh, I had a long discussion with our Anesthesia Department chairman, Peter Winter. We decided that I should resign as chief and he appointed Jim Snyder as the new division chief. I had tenure as a full professor since 1975 and could continue my career on the CCM faculty. In 1995, I was promoted to distinguished service professor of CCM.

CCM Recruitment

When the position as chairman of our Department of Surgery unexpectedly became available, Mitchel Fink was one of the prominent candidates. As a most reputable surgeon at Boston University well known for his extensive CCM research, he was offered and accepted the simultaneously vacated position as chief of our Division of CCM. He quickly moved our division forward by promoting clinical and basic research. He also established much improved financial conditions. Peter Safar and I had applied twice in the 1980s for a separate department of CCM but turned down by the Medical School Executive Committee, since the CCM Division was not considered financially secure without protection by an existing department. This was now different and Mitch Fink was encouraged to try again. Thus, the first American CCM Department was established at the University of Pittsburgh. Mitch Fink was appointed as the founding chairman. During his reign an endowed Grenvik chair in CCM was approved after successful fundraising. An annual Grenvik lecture was introduced in the CCM Department in 2003 and similarly at the annual SCCM congresses from 2009.

In 1996 when giving an invited lecture at the Royal Infirmary of Glasgow in Scotland, ICU director, Ian McA Ledingham, introduced me to Derek Angus, an internist, his best ICU physician trainee. Derek Angus wanted further CCM training in the USA. So I invited him to become a fellow in our training program in the upcoming academic year. After an impressive year of clinical training, he stayed on as a research fellow at the Safar Center for Resuscitation Research under Patrick Kochanek's leadership. Because of his outstanding performance, he was then offered a faculty position and escalated quickly on his career ladder. When Mitch Fink resigned as CCM chairman to start a private pharmaceutical company, Derek Angus was appointed the new chairman in very strong competition. The young CCM Department continued to grow rapidly with very large NIH and other federal research grants. The most active researchers in addition to Derek Angus included Michael Pinsky, John Kellum, Patrick Kochanek, and Ann Thompson.

Retirement Problems

My involvement in CCM during these years was only at half time. Because of nationwide economical restraints, in 2008 the dean of our medical school requested that all departments should reduce their current budgets by 5 % and another 5 % in the following academic year. I offered to have my salary decreased immediately by 5 % but was told that savings should not be done by salary reduction but rather through decrease in the number of positions. As the oldest CCM faculty member at the time, I was asked to resign. With tenure, I could not be fired. I talked it over with my wife Inger who had suffered a severe stroke in 2003 which left her with a left sided hemiplegia. Initially, she could walk with a cane and as a right-handed person she never lost her ability to speak. But she gradually deteriorated and became increasingly dependent on her wheelchair. I was needed more frequently for her support. We had a home caregiver every weekday, but during evenings, nights, and weekends, I was the caregiver. So it had become obvious that I could not continue my part-time work. Therefore, I agreed with our current CCM Department chairman, Derek Angus, to resign and retire at age 80 from July 1, 2009.

In September that year, my long-term colleagues and friends, Michael Pinsky and John Hoyt, on behalf of our CCM Department organized an outstanding farewell party. Michael Pinsky announced that I had been promoted to retirement as distinguished professor emeritus of CCM. Other speakers included the Dean, Senior Vice Chancellor Arthur Levine. The current SCCM president spoke for this society and Sten Rubertsson, MD, PhD, represented the University of Uppsala in Sweden.

We remained in our Upper St Clair house in Pittsburgh for another 5 years. Our annual visits to Sweden were discontinued as we could no longer travel with Inger by air. But we had a large motor home, and although it was difficult to get Inger on board, once inside, it was spacious enough to wheel her around in the wheelchair. So we made several weekend trips and one longer trip each year. With bedroom, toilet, shower, and kitchen in the RV, it was a very practical way to travel with Inger.

Our son Anders was both the driver and cook. We pulled our little Honda Fit behind like a dingy, using it for short sightseeing trips. Inger enjoyed these excursions. We visited the beautiful national parks out West. The last trip was in 2014 which took us to the Canadian Atlantic Coast. But in early 2015, Inger suddenly deteriorated with aspiration problems and developed severe dyspnea which ended her life on January 21 at age 82. After a most memorable funeral, she was buried in Pittsburgh at the Forest Lawn Garden, next to our long deceased son Christer.

Leaving Pittsburgh

I started to supervise a thorough renovation of our old home as I prepared to leave Pittsburgh. But in late February, living alone in our house, I woke up on the floor one night, unable to get up. Both my legs were paralyzed and painful. Our youngest son Stefan as a thoughtful physician had seen to it that I was equipped with an alarm system which probably saved my life this night. I pushed the alarm button and within a few minutes first a police car showed up with two officers and shortly thereafter an ambulance with two paramedics. The seriousness of my condition was recognized and I was promptly transported to nearby St Clair Hospital. I discussed my problem with the emergency medicine physician on call in the ED. Sky high CPK values along with dark brown urine made it clear that I was suffering from rhabdomyolysis. I had taken Lipitor for many years and rhabdomyolysis is a serious, well-known side effect of that statin, so it was immediately discontinued. Large volumes of intravenous fluid administration saved my kidneys and muscle function began to return to my legs which were enormously edematous, indicating use of diuretics., After a week, I could stand up and walk with a walker. Following another week in a rehabilitation center, I could return home and continue supervising the ongoing renovation of our house. It took 3 months and was very expensive but did the trick. The house sold in 2 weeks after it was put on the market.

Retiring in Texas

I was offered and accepted an invitation to join our daughter Monica and her husband Michael McGinley in Houston. Their children had long since left the parents' large house. Anders drove me down to Texas in his roomy SUV, with enough space to take my few remaining belongings. Monica and Mike arranged for me to sleep in their large master bedroom with attached bathroom on the first floor, since I could not walk up the stairs. With a pool in the backyard, I have tried to swim twice a day, 500 m each time for a total of 1,000 m per day. Since I can no longer walk very well, the daily swimming has contributed greatly to my recovery. But half a year after my rhabdomyolysis attack, I still did not have normal sensation in my feet. I walk with a quad cane for support and no longer drive by myself. Monica takes me around in her van and pushes me as needed in the wheelchair I inherited from Inger.

Over the Thanksgiving holidays in 2015, I spent 2 weeks with my youngest son Stefan in Bristol, TN. He is divorced and lives with Amber, a most attractive young woman. His two daughters no longer live at home, both attending college at this time. When the 2 weeks were up, I returned to Houston in time for Christmas celebration but without Inger for the first time. She is greatly missed by all of us.

In conclusion, I live a good retirement life in Texas and am well taken care of by my children.

Important lessons learned and exemplified in this chapter:

1. Cure of depression is not accomplished with drugs and sick leave.
2. Finding and eliminating the cause of depression are the key to cure.
3. Successful medical career is based on interest, enthusiasm, and unique qualifications in a rapidly growing new field with eminent positions in high demand.
4. A high academic position is not reached without thorough education and scientific research.
5. Pediatric and adult CCM training do not mix.
6. Specialty board exams are essential for success.
7. Each new specialty needs a scientific journal.
8. In CCM close cooperation important by physicians with nurses and other health-care professionals.
9. Use every opportunity to involve government.
10. Keep up with crucial development.
11. Publish important observations and research findings.
12. Not the inventor but rather the publisher gets the credit for a new technique calling it to professional attention.
13. Develop and introduce new systems such as use of rapid response teams.
14. Use alarm systems for invalids and elderly.
15. Use wheelchairs and other suitable devices for invalids and elderly.
16. Frequent physical exercise promotes cardiopulmonary function.
17. Exercise the brain through reading and writing.
18. If healthy, elderly academicians can contribute significantly into their 80s through nonclinical involvement, such as administration, teaching, research, and publication.

References

1. Grenvik A. Respiratory, circulatory and metabolic effects of respirator treatment. Acta Anaestesiologica Scandinavica, Supplement 19, 1966.
2. Grenvik A. Role of allied health professionals in critical care medicine. Crit Care Med. 1974;2:6–10.

3. Grenvik A. Certification of special competence in critical care medicine as a new subspecialty. A status report. Crit Care Med. 1979;6:355–9.
4. Grenvik A, Leonard JJ, Arens JF, Carey LC, Disney FA. Critical care medicine. Certification as a multidisciplinary subspecialty. Crit Care Med. 1981;9:117–25.
5. Grenvik A, Ayres S, Holbrook P, Shoemaker W. Textbook of critical care. 4th ed. Philadelphia: WB Saunders; 2000.

Chapter 5
Transitions from the Academic Heap: New Directions Within the System

James V. Snyder

I practiced in a golden age of physiology. We built on an age of resuscitation, and medicine had not yet become molecular. I joined Peter Safar's world and was paid to work in the ICU, under Ake Grenvik's supervision, as resident, fellow, and junior staff. Our explication of the physiology to resolve opposing viewpoints gained us authority and led to publications that rationalized promotion. Getting authority also required physical presence when the admitting physicians came to visit, which cost time at home.

The critical care division grew rapidly as ICU capacity expanded from 16 to 120 beds. Consultation with Margaret Schaffer and a retreat to assess strengths, weaknesses, opportunities, and threats (SWOT) led to a restructured Critical Care Division. The organization allowed Ake to step down, and at Ake's recommendation, Peter Winter designated me to replace him as chief.

For the first 5 years, I recruited physicians from other centers and matched their skills with the needs of our growing specialty programs. Luke Chelluri and then Arthur Boujoukos kept order on the clinical side. David Powner developed a structured educational program, and Paul Rogers developed the medical student exposure to become a required rotation. Michael Pinsky assured our insight to bedside physiology. Life was good those first 5 years. The second five, not so much.

Managed care changed everything. Costs had to be controlled, and the "expensive care units" were obvious targets. System-wide fiscal responsibility was not in the job description. Neither the docs nor the organization were prepared for the constraints and requirements thrust upon us. We were pressed to reduce costs by stretching coverage and reducing chargeable care; quality of coding to maximize revenue competed with concern for quality of care. Marc Roberts explained how the beast had become so ugly *(Your Money or Your Life)*. Mini-executive MBA courses helped us morph toward our new roles. The Institute for Healthcare Improvement

J.V. Snyder, MD
Critical Care Medicine, University of Pittsburgh Medical Center, Pittsburgh, PA, USA
e-mail: snyderjv@me.com

© Springer International Publishing Switzerland 2016
D. Crippen (ed.), *The Intensivist's Challenge: Aging and Career Growth in a High-Stress Medical Specialty*, DOI 10.1007/978-3-319-30454-0_5

promoted a collaborative approach to changing the system, and the Advisory Board Company provided best practices in difficult areas, such as aligning incentives with productivity. But UPMC wasn't interested in the IHI approach, and the fact that I had not negotiated for financial control became a serious constriction. Our efforts within the division, especially by Mary Beth Coleman and Arthur Boujoukos, reduced labs up to 60 % and length of stay by a third without cost in outcome, but I was not able to have these savings recognized in the critical care balance sheet. Division research funding increased by $2 million on my watch, but I had no direct role and inadequate experience in funded research to catalyze further. The division had great strengths, but I was not prepared to lead it through this adaptive phase, and I stepped down to make room for a better skill set. Chairman Len Firestone made a most constructive contribution in recruiting Mitchell Fink as division chief. Mitch developed areas I could not and led us to become the first independent department of CCM in an academic center.

It was an error not to negotiate my post-chief role and compensation. I felt unprepared to take on a full service, and instead I attempted a self-funded return to brain research. Ake and I reduced our footprint by moving into the same office. With paid time less than 50 %, I required a provost's exemption to retain tenure, which I would need to get post-retirement health-care insurance.

The research effort, supported by the Laerdal Company and Drs. Keith Theilborn and Howard Yonas, yielded results that were intriguing, but not enough to fund this 7th decade researcher absent a recent track record. Pitt's health insurance offer to the over 65 faculty induced my retirement from that half of my job, and I returned to night calls for clinical income. Fortunately that was a pleasure, as my residual skills especially suited bedside support of fellows in emergent evaluations. Those long hours became tiring enough to retire in my 39th year at Pitt, with a retirement cache that should be quite adequate if nurtured more carefully than I would prefer.

Knowing How the Brain Works Is Helpful to Getting the Big Picture

Two insights on brain function have provided fresh perspective. Seeing how neuroplasticity can be manipulated reveals the power of the mind to cause and relieve disease and so invites mind-body thinking into clinical practice and into aging well [1].

The familiar blind spot exemplifies a brain mechanism behind our failure to see what can later seem so obvious. It is a hard-wired process whereby the brain draws firm conclusions *automatically* from whatever observations it has already accepted [2]. The visual blind spot is an excellent example, where the blank area is filled in, instantly, based on the surrounding visual field. Learning is resisted and conclusions are rejected *without thought*, unless supported by a substantial field of previously accepted data or by a direct experience. Instead we back up our intuitive conclusion with reams of *found rather than sound* evidence.

This automated process can explain our experimental bias, political blindness, and combative theologies.

In spiritual matters, our cultural acceptance of Descartes' recommendation to respect conclusions in proportion to their reproducibility caused us to disparage uncontrolled observations, hence anything from "across the veil." Yet quantum mechanics informs a complete lack of control in most of the energy-mass we know exists. Edgar Cayce's work provides a more credible and relevant perspective than do established religions [3, 4].

Airway and Breathing

My peri-retirement professional occupation has been in the A and B of resuscitation. For most of my career, I taught in an annual cadaver airway lab to prepare airway novices to serve as first responders to codes. Our airway-novice[1] fellows now report that after training only in our lab, they are successful in 93 % in their (supervised) management of the airway in critically ill patients. That program has roots throughout my career, so an accounting fits the theme of this book.

In short, advanced airway skills I learned in the Navy enabled safe and effective training of airway-novice[1] fellows in codes, which provided a rich feedback to modify our cadaver airway lab. Modification of cadavers to simulate spontaneous breathing proved effective to teach noninvasive management. Dissection provided fresh insights on epiglottis control and on why elevating the head improves exposure in difficult intubations. Our program is outlined below, followed by notes on its career-related roots. My partner Dr. Steve Orebaugh and I hope that the program can be verified and exported, and we invite critical reflection (thoughtthatcounts73@gmail.com).

Summary of the Current Program on Bag-Mask Ventilation

Trainees learn the "feel of the bag" from pressure-flow patterns generated by manually driven bellows. Then, using "spontaneously" breathing cadavers (Fig. 5.1), the fellows learn to keep the mouth open under the mask, balanced by gentle lift behind the rami. They use "seal-seeking" pressure oscillation to instantly assess and monitor mask seal and manual CPAP to splint the upper and lower airway. A drop in bag pressure with patient inspiration confirms airway patency and assures synchronous assisted ventilation. Changes in effective compliance help them detect

---

[1] Airway novice is defined as pre-lab intubation experience less than 10 intubations.

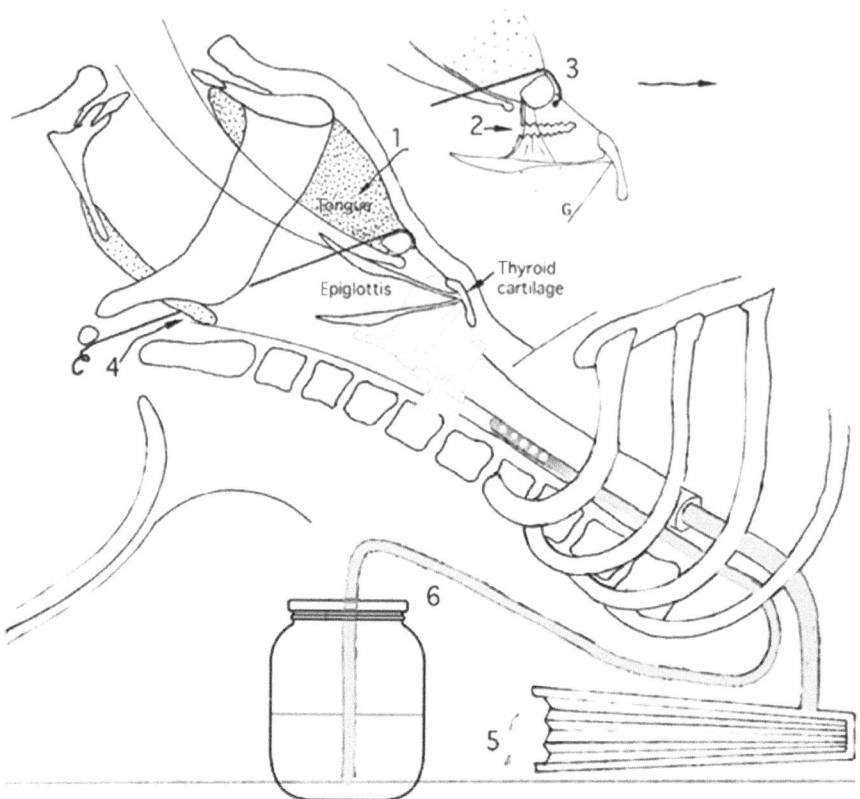

Fig. 5.1 Cadaver airway training model. *1.* Tongue bulk and response is maintained by injection of tissue building gel. *2.* The glossoepiglottic membrane is incised to allow the epiglottis to lie in its normal position shadowing the glottis. *3.* Ease of laryngeal exposure is controlled by a surrogate for the stylohyoid ligament: wire passed behind the anterior thyrohyoid ligament and anterior to the hyoid body, past the lesser cornu to exit behind the ear lobe on each side. *4.* The soft palate is injected with saline to simulate expiratory flap valve obstruction during mask ventilation. *5.* Spontaneous ventilation is simulated by lifting a bellows attached to an endotracheal tube passed retrograde via the bronchus intermedius, after lobectomy. *6.* The effects of upper airway pressure and maneuvers and of cricoid pressure on esophageal insufflation are manifest by air passing into a nasogastric tube inserted retrograde to a level below the cricopharyngeus, with its distal end placed in a bottle of soapy water. Gastric insufflation is represented by foaming within the bottle at the bedside. The tube also allows simulation of regurgitation or emesis during laryngoscopy. *G*: glottis opening [5]. (Reproduced from Anaesthesia and Intensive Care with the kind permission of the Australian Society of Anaesthetists)

changes in upper and lower airway obstruction, "chest wall" compliance, or mask seal and to distinguish whether airway obstruction is expiratory or inspiratory.

NG tubes inserted retrograde to below the upper esophageal sphincter in fresh cadavers allows trainees to experience need for and proper application of cricoid pressure (CP). With the external end of the NG tube in a bottle of soapy water, they can confirm the usual resistance to GI before the upper sphincter has been opened and the ease of inducing GI after the sphincter has been opened by high pressure.

They see that GI usually stops with only light pressure on the cricoid, but that GI is increased with head tilt and jaw thrust, requiring higher CP. The experience encourages routine CP with the triple airway maneuver.

The NG tube also simulates emesis, hence opportunity to demonstrate the ineffectiveness of routine practices such as turning the patient's head and suctioning and how within seconds a very large patient can be turned past full lateral to drain the oropharynx and then how to perform BMV and DL in the lateral position – all as taught by Dr. George D. Mitchell (see below).

Direct Laryngoscopy

Thorough, stress-free familiarization with laryngoscopic anatomy is the first priority in DL training. Detailed videos of the operator's view precede the lab. The cadavers are ideally positioned in near-maximal head elevation to allow delicate bimanual manipulation using conventionally shaped blades, with blade-based video for instructor feedback.

Maneuvers are taught separately, including ramp construction, precise control of the epiglottis, maximal use of assistants from the beginning of the procedure until head elevation is maximal or exposure ideal, and early use of external laryngeal manipulation. Then these steps are integrated into one smooth sequence, and that sequence is reduced to less than 30 s. Fellows are advised to seek maximal exposure in every case, to ensure adequate exposure in the most difficult case.

The most important of the specific maneuvers is the "epi flip." The blade-based video feed informs how pressing the blade tip against the upper part of the midline suspension ligament of the epiglottis – the "sweet spot" – gives better exposure with less force than does placement in the vallecula [6]. Advancing the blade tip as little as 2 mm flips the epiglottis up from shadowing the glottis to flat against the blade, out of sight, with no vertical lift required. The "sweet spot" is not visible by DL, so the critical next step is to learn how to find that "sweet spot" when the operator can see only the tip of the epiglottis. Learning how tissues proximate to the sweet spot respond to small pulses of blade tip pressure informs how to reposition the blade.

Trainees then experience how lowering the head impairs the ability both to lift the epiglottis and to expose the glottis, then that most of the force required in DL is for axial manipulation, and finally that well-directed assistance can strikingly reduce the operator's gross effort and improve their precision and success. To test trainee understanding of axial manipulation and command of assistants, we increase tension on the surrogate stylohyoid ligament until exposure requires considerable effort. They are expected to direct the assistants' force, including caudad pressure on the vertex, to achieve "walkaway" assistance: in which they need only a light touch to gain optimal exposure and can remove the blade, "walk away," return, and regain the same easy exposure, all while the assistants work hard to maintain that position.

Two hours of one-on-one training at five stations with fresh cadavers enables most novices to achieve maximal exposure using the complete integrated sequence within 30 s. Our novices report their remarkable performance after a total of three and a half hours in two sessions, an hour of lecture/discussion, and thereafter only bedside training. OR rotation for airway experience is no longer routine.

Validation and Export

The program's success has led to less than satisfactory compromise. We have been mandated to use "light preservation" techniques rather than fresh cadavers, because training our fellows, new faculty, and trainees from other programs required use of fresh cadavers for longer than is esthetically appropriate. Even light preservation technique reduces authenticity of important features. The soft palate is less likely to act as a flap valve; the tongue doesn't slur against the posterior pharyngeal wall, so jaw thrust is no longer required to keep the pharynx open; and the epiglottis is more likely to be lifted with the tongue than to remain hanging over the glottis. We perform further modifications to compensate, as by injecting the soft palate and tongue and sectioning the glossoepiglottic membrane to allow the epiglottis to drop, but cannot fully restore authenticity of tissue response.

Use of preservation makes it difficult to achieve the validation that one would hope to find before export of this program is attempted. Patient risk and informed consent issues impair use of stable patients in the OR for most of this training. Validation and export will require a condensed program using fresh cadavers, until authentic dry lab simulation can be developed.

Personal Roots of the Airway Management Program

Near-drowning might have seeded my interest. I was four. I remember the riptide current, choking, my arms going limp, and looking up through light green water, fading to black. Safar hadn't yet described advanced airway techniques [7, 8] but dad was an ENT doc. I regained consciousness and got to eat lemon-lime sherbet.

I signed on to an anesthesia support training program in the Navy after internship, to avoid a prolonged hitch as an untrained GP. After a year with Drs. Jerry Phelps and Bill Owens, I was paired for 2 years with Dr. George D. Mitchell, who sent me to a Safar conference. Safar's focus on brain resuscitation and intensive care pulled me from internal medicine to anesthesiology.

Dr. Mitchell was an extraordinary teacher. In most cases he had me use bag and mask rather than intubation and constant observation – an ear to a pretracheal or esophageal stethoscope, a hand on the latex anesthesia bag, and an eye on the procedure. Safar's triple airway maneuver (head tilt, mouth open under the mask, and jaw thrust) was routine.

Keeping the mouth open avoids expiratory obstruction from the soft palate acting as a flap valve. And jaw thrust, in addition to holding the tongue forward, prevents complete ball-valve obstruction due to the epiglottis dropping over and sealing the glottis [9].

Mitchell had me bag by feel rather than by eye. The least drop in pressure with patient inspiration confirmed airway patency, and synchronized assistance is almost reflexive. A hand on the bag informs mask fit, airway patency, patient effort, and static and effective compliance. The resting hand also assures manual CPAP, which eliminates or reduces inspiratory and expiratory stridor and splints open the pharynx and even the edematous post-extubation glottis [9–11].

Manually controlling lung volume and excursion gave thoracic surgeons optimal advantage and gave me hours observing closing capacity, resorption atelectasis, and the effectiveness and safety of prolonged low pressure to recruit atelectic lung.

"Feel of the bag" technique became routine in the Maryland Shock Trauma Unit when McAslan brought latex anesthesia bags from the OR to recruit atelectic lung (personal observation). The flexible Laerdal bags in use at UPMC provided much the same feel. Addition of a pressure T between the tube and bag allowed manual control of end-expiratory pressure and aided study of pulmonary stabilization and recruitment [12–14]. The currently available disposable bags are less sensitive, but by flexing the bag, *most novices can still quickly learn the technique.* CPAP and bagging by feel along with the triple airway maneuver can establish high SpO2 before and between laryngoscopy attempts in almost every case.

Our use of "informed" cricoid pressure (CP) came from both clinical and lab experience. Although Greenbaum had confirmed mask CPAP could be applied long term without GI [15], GI was common in codes. Head tilt and jaw thrust that are required to open the airway tend to pull open the piriform recess. First responders are taught, correctly, that airway pressure greater than 40 cm H2O may be necessary because airway obstruction may not be fully relieved by the triple airway maneuver. That high pressure may be necessary sometimes, when the airway can't be maintained by best technique, resulting in frequent use to try to compensate for suboptimal technique. High airway pressure from a first responder's effort can elevate gastric pressure above the opening pressures of the esophageal sphincters and inflate the esophagus into an open conduit.

An additional cause of GI is when airway managers (including some quite experienced) misinterpret the rocking movement of dyspneic patients, due to asynchronous respiratory effort, and squeeze the bag exactly out of sequence. Feel of the bag avoids that error.

Roots of Direct Laryngoscopy Techniques

Our program became multidisciplinary about the same time as I joined, and suddenly half our trainees were airway novices. They were expected to manage the airway in codes, assisted by respiratory therapists, until an airway expert could respond, and we were expected to give them airway skills with an annual experience of only about 50 cases. OR training was limited by capacity and was oriented to basic techniques rather than emergent care. We needed a shorter learning curve. Bedside performance and the cadaver lab were both improved by 30 plus years of feedback.

We credit Levitan for initiating DL as a science [16]. His doubling of novice initial success rate by showing videos of the operator's view of the larynx [17] led to our emphasis on advance video study and advocacy to teach DL using conventionally shaped blades with a video feed (Karl Storz, Verathon).

Levitan's emphasis on optimal technique in the first attempt increased our focus on immediate training in advanced technique rather than basic [15]. Dr. David Huang referred us to new studies on head elevation [18, 19], which led us to understand that mobilization of the airway skeleton is controlled by a strutted cable suspension system – the styloid process, stylohyoid ligament, and hyoid bone – whereby lifting the head converts the hyoid from a dorsally secured strut to a forward-swinging trapeze. We routinely duplicate this mechanism by inserting a wire in place of the stylohyoid ligament, vary tension on the wire to control difficulty, and relieve difficulty by head elevation.

Validation and export of the program have been inhibited by inadequate description and difficulty in reproducing the model. We plan to move on those fronts and invite challenge and collaboration (thoughtthatcounts73@gmail.com).

References

1. Doidge N. The brain's way of healing: remarkable discoveries and recoveries from the frontiers of neuroplasticity. New York: Viking Penguins; 2015.
2. Ramachandran VS, Blakeslee S. Phantoms in the brain. New York: Quill; 1999.
3. Kirkpatrick S. Edgar Cayce: an American Prophet. New York: Riverhead Books; 2001.
4. Todeschi KJ, Reed H. Contemporary Cayce: a complete exploration using today's philosophy and science. Virginia Beach: VA: ARE Press; 2014.
5. Wise EM, Henao JP, Gomez H, Snyder§ J, Roolf P, Orebaugh SL. The impact of a cadaver-based airway lab on critical care fellows' direct laryngoscopy skills published in Anaesth Intensive Care V 2015;43:2.
6. Fink BR, Demarest RJ. Laryngeal biomechanics. Cambridge: Harvard University Press; 1978. The text refers to blade placement in the vallecula but positioning against the epiglottis suspension ligament is diagrammed in figure 8.4.
7. Safar P, Escarraga LA, Elam JO. A comparison of the mouth-to-mouth and mouth-to-airway methods of artificial respiration with the chest-pressure arm-lift methods. N Engl J Med. 1958;258:671–7.
8. Safar P, Escarraga LA, Chang F. Upper airway obstruction in the unconscious patient. J Appl Physiol. 1959;14:760–4.
9. Fink BR. The etiology and treatment of laryngeal spasm. Anesthesiology. 1956;569–577.
10. Hillman DR, Walsh JH, Maddison KJ, et al. Evolution of changes in upper airway collapsibility during slow induction of anesthesia with propofol. Anesthesiology. 2009;111:63–71.
11. Schwab RJ. Radiographic imaging in the diagnostic evaluation of sleep apnea patients. UpToDate Version. 2005.
12. Semmes EJ, Tobin MJ, Snyder JV, Grenvik A. Subjective and objective measurement of tidal volume in critically Ill patients. Chest. 1985;87:577–9.
13. Novak RA, Snyder JV, Shumaker L, Pinsky MR. Periodic hyperinflation improve Gas exchange in patients with hypoxemic respiratory failure. Crit Care Med. 1987;15(12):1081–5.

14. Scholton DJ, Novak R, Snyder JV. Directed manual recruitment of collapsed lung in intubated and nonintubated patients. Am Surg. 1985;51:330–5.
15. Greenbaum DM, Snyder JV, Grenvik A. Continuous positive airway pressure without tracheal intubation in spontaneously breathing patients. Chest. 1976;69:615–20.
16. Levitan RM. The importance of a laryngoscopy strategy and optimal conditions in emergency intubation. Anesth Analg. 2005;100:899–900.
17. Levitan RM, Goldman TS, Bryon DA, et al. Training with video imaging improves the initial intubation success rates of paramedic trainees in an operating room setting. Ann Emerg Med. 2001;37:46–50.
18. Levitan RM, Mechem CC, Ochroch EA, Shofer FS, Hollander JE. Head-elevated laryngoscopy position: improving laryngeal exposure during laryngoscopy by increasing head elevation. Ann Emerg Med. 2003;41:322–30.
19. Schmitt HJ, Mang H. Head and neck elevation beyond the sniffing position improves laryngeal view in cases of difficult direct laryngoscopy. J Clin Anesth. 2002;14:335–8.

Chapter 6
The Ageing Intensivist and Global Medical Politics

Richard Burrows

> *"Youth, which is forgiven everything, forgives itself nothing:*
> *age which forgives itself everything, is forgiven nothing".*
>
> *George Bernard Shaw Preface Man and Superman:*
> *Maxims for Revolutionists.*

As one ages it becomes easy to sympathize with those who forget to replace the petrol cap and easy also to read the maxim above and understand why older individuals are viewed with a critical eye in respect of responsibilities for difficult decisions. Associating, as cause and effect, problems and the fact of ageing is, however, not as simple as a maxim that generalizes human behaviour. Also even though there is deterioration with age, it is not clear whether problems generated by the hubris of youth are any less of a problem. Experience leads one to beware of certain situations [1] that a more youthful individual would tackle without due thought. Also there are a number of other reasons why performance should fail other than age in particular dependency on alcohol or other drugs. The problem then is deteriorating performance rather than, specifically, age and how society should deal with the underperforming clinician.

Society is a complex system that evolves over time whereby individuals who are themselves complex interact with this complex system. Attempts to render the "system" down to more simple models are fraught with difficulties. Religious or secular moral systems each construct their own ethical arguments based on moral values that are specific to their own interpretation of their particular moral code. Then, by their own interpretation of right or wrong, they proselytize in an attempt to force their own moral point [2], and although the ethical arguments of non-malfeasance, justice, autonomy and primum non nocere are, prima facie, indisputable, the underlying moral values can be quite contrary to the argued ethical point. This, in turn, leads to conflict particularly in difficult issues of end of life or abortion as lack of tolerance rapidly gains tenure. Individual actions are judged against the background of the system and may be lauded or condemned in equal

R. Burrows, MD
Private Practice Bon Secours Hospital, Galway, Ireland
e-mail: sworrub@gmail.com

© Springer International Publishing Switzerland 2016
D. Crippen (ed.), *The Intensivist's Challenge: Aging and Career Growth in a High-Stress Medical Specialty*, DOI 10.1007/978-3-319-30454-0_6

measure with an outcome depending on who is doing the judging [3]. Moral attitudes or cultures differ from place to place and the differences can be substantial and sometimes even abhorrent to the individual (and vice versa) when he/she sees individuals being treated contrary to their own particular moral makeup. Furthermore any difficult decision will be accompanied by consequences that can only be judged in hindsight. The consequences of a particular action under such circumstances may be viewed such as to ensure the a priori behaviour of the individual matches the culture wherein he practices to the point that, as stated by Shaw [4] – "…it may be said that the assent of the majority is the only sanction known to *ethics*". Then again the individual's personal belief may well be in step with the culture of the time – which will keep him out of trouble as long as the system doesn't change under his feet! The "systems" are complex indeed!

Anecdote is not science, but then much of medical science is little more than a controlled series of repeatable anecdotes and, in the words of Poincaré – "Sociology is the science with the greatest number of methods and the least results". But then 40 years ago, embarking on a medical career, we didn't really see that as we seemed to be on the cusp of a technological revolution that would eventually address all problems. The heart had been transplanted just a few years earlier and renal transplantation was a regular occurrence. Advances were so obvious that statistical analysis hardly seemed necessary, exemplified by a 50 % reduction in mortality by the use of ventilation in tetanus neonatorum [5] Antibiotics were introduced with minimal research demanded of today's drugs.

Technology is only part of a complex whole but it has contributed enormously to sociological and clinical problems of an ethical nature that, unlike moral systems, cannot be the subject of research.

Clinically, many questions quickly became intractable – what is the best fluid for resuscitation in trauma? And how much? Do steroids work? In what dosage? How long should we ventilate? What's the best inotrope? Are antibiotics really indicated? Why are there new drugs that are later withdrawn? Various treatments are often controversial and are based on the notion of "best medical evidence", but medical evidence is often highly questionable and biased [6] to the point of fraud [7] and also such that an author can ask how much of the science is of a zombie nature seemingly alive only because of an apparent limitless amount of funds [8]. Such are the rewards for medical research that problems of fabrication, plagiarism and other forms of fraud are far from uncommon [9].

There was another even more intractable side in that there were questions of a social, ethical and economic nature that were temporized as questions that would be answered if not now then surely the near future would bring answers. Instead the problems became more intractable and with a little examination were even seen to be questions that had been be addressed in antiquity by individuals such as Plato and more recently by Shaw in his prologue to "The Doctor's Dilemma" – "In legislation and social organization, proceed on the principle that invalids, meaning persons who cannot keep themselves alive by their own activities, cannot, beyond reason, expect to be kept alive by the activity of others. There is a point at which the most energetic policeman or doctor, when called upon to deal with an apparently drowned person, gives up artificial respiration, although it is never possible to declare with certainty, at any point short of decomposition, that another 5 min of the exercise would not effect resuscitation. The theory that every individual alive is of infinite value is legislatively impracticable" [4]. Clearly the main problem was not how to treat but rather when to treat or when to stop treatment. Over the years technology has only made these questions more difficult as society and clinicians have grappled with them.

There are other issues too. As we introduce new techniques or machinery, we introduce new problems [3]. There was no such thing as a ventilator disconnect before the introduction of ventilators and likewise cardiopulmonary bypass, induced hypothermia, dialysis and so on. Technology therefore comes with risk as well as benefit.

Legal attitudes are also fluid, and although law is different in different countries with different systems and cultures, all systems are essentially adversarial with varying burdens of proof all leaning towards the hegemony of autonomy [10] that brutally overwhelms other voices in medical ethics debates. This means that in the western world at least there is confusion as to whether medical mishaps should be judged according to a civil or criminal standard [11, 12], This is complicated by the fact that all medical mishaps are looked at with the benefit of hindsight. The clinician who has lost a patient is at the mercy of a justice system that can be biased simply by a bad outcome [3, 13].

Science, if it depends on anything, depends on rigid definitions such as the speed of light or, for example, the coefficient of expansion of copper that holds absolutely true within certain parameters. Outside the parameters the definitions fail as when the copper melts. Within the parameters the definition is immutable, unchangeable and extremely useful as such definitions of the coefficient of expansion of two different metals allow us to measure temperature or allow controlled expansion for a vapour contributing the safety of anaesthesia. The social sciences, on the other hand, are anything but rigid. Instead, definitions are based on the mathematics of probability with principles that are often sufficiently vague as to be dependent on the opinion of experts who, in turn, are, themselves, influenced by questions of culture, political dispensation, religion, selfishness, greed and/or economic expediency. Granted this is countered by altruism, simple decency and guilt at the plight of fellow man and so on but either way it is bias none the less. Furthermore a decision based on probability carries with it the propensity to be wrong in spite of best efforts to reduce the risk. And worse, these decisions invariably incorporate abstract, indefinable terms such as "quality" [14] and "fairness" which makes them similar to the mathematical equivalent of division/multiplication by zero or infinity! They are then definitions dependent on the observer's notion of "fairness" or "quality". We think we reason but thought too is "always rooted in values and motivations. "We think not for the sake of thinking but to achieve certain goals based on our system of values" [15]. This, in turn, means that autonomy becomes little more than a statement of wants rather than needs and expressed by individuals exhibiting little other than an intense fear of death and evidenced by the fact that 62 % of bankruptcies in the United States are by reason of medical debts [16] and that those with insight – i.e. doctors choose to die in bed! [17].

The World Health Authority defines health as "a state of complete physical, mental and social well-being and not merely the absence of disease or infirmity" [18]. This is a decision that has not been changed since 1948 presumably because no group of experts has been able to develop a more obtuse definition. Since 1948 there have been enormous changes in technology together with an unimpeachable emphasis on autonomy.

This is not to say there have been no advances in medical science. There have been advances, often wonderfully so. Many cancers now seem to be little more than chronic diseases. Transplantation extends to new boundaries regularly and the science of prosthetic surgery has advanced to the point that was science fiction in the recent past.

The downside is that as technology has come with an economic cost that has outstripped the ability of all but the wealthiest to pay for it. Those of lesser wealth must depend on some third party or government insurance. The Tragedy of the commons [19] and a perfect storm of a technological imperative, culture of autonomy and fear of death [20] have often meant little more than an insistence by the patient or other interested groups on prolonged, inappropriate life support in many cases [21, 22]. Under the circumstances it takes little scrutiny to understand how such issues as quality of life and economic expediency rapidly become quite inapposite, manipulated by clinicians, administrators and politicians alike – each unable to deal with the situation as economic reality squares up to abstract clinical credulity in the face of unrestricted patient demand.

In dealing with this problem of inappropriate use of technology in the face of economic reality, there is the doublespeak of administrators and politicians who would have the populace believe all is well while, in intensive care at any rate, clinicians are telling them that there are not the beds to deal with a tenth of the patients presented for treatment. It was bad enough, in this part of the world, when medical matters were controlled by a political system ideologically driven to classify people according to colour, but when that noxious system failed, as it was programmed to fail by the unassailable power of the majority, it was replaced by a system that quickly showed itself to be little more than a thin patina of democracy spread over corruption of the first order. The upshot was that budgets were even more curtailed to the point that the unit was closed and the hospital found itself more strained than ever to supply even basic care. All this is in the face of nearly ten thousand vacancies in the system while there are nearly four applicants for every post [23] Unfortunately, one anathema has simply replaced another anathema. Discussions with colleagues around the world taught me that others in other parts of the world were not really interested in our problems but mention Obamacare or the NHS! It quickly becomes clear that the problems are the same – the economic difficulties are the same but different cultures deal with the problems in their own way.

Under these circumstances the individual who is at odds with the system can find himself on thin ice.

It is difficult to ascertain the number of ICU beds necessary to service a particular population. One group [24] came to a figure of 21 beds per 100,000 people. At the time that paper was published, the number of critical care beds in KwaZulu-

Natal was less than 1.5/100,000 and that was for all disciplines including paediatrics. Under the circumstances, the only rational mechanism to deal with the problems was to make decisions based on the probability of survival: triage. As a coping mechanism, I found it easier and easier to triage those with chronic disease – particularly if they had been accorded a "good innings". The notion that they were unlikely to survive was the cornerstone for the decision-making process.

At this point it is important to understand what a decision is and why it can be wrong. A decision is a deliberate choice between options of varying probabilities and in respect of this it should be clear that a decision based on certainty is not a decision at all it is merely an acceptance of circumstances as outlined in Shaw's *point of decomposition* above [4]. There is a simple statistical propensity to be wrong without any bias or negligence. There is more in as much as the individual making the decision is himself given to make a decision based on his own biases and pressures that will hopefully be in keeping with the *zeitgeist*. That said, by far the commonest reason not to admit was that the unit was full. 50 % of patients were refused admission the reasons being one of the three: (1) the unit was full, (2) the admission would be futile or (3) the patient could be safely handled on the ward. By far the main reason was the unit was full. It has to be said that for those working in the unit, it was easier to refuse admission on the basis that the unit was full rather than enter into what sometimes turned into snarling confrontations with colleagues as intensive care could do nothing for the patient. Clearly, when colleagues are working together, the conversations are often simplified to avoid confronting any "big questions" and to merely get through the day, no morality, just expediency dictated by the demands and expectations of the moment. It meant that the stresses were such that, in order to avoid many of the confrontations, patients were still admitted against better judgment and, in turn, that still meant a 50 % mortality of admitted patients and a consequent destruction of morale. I drew comfort from the fact that similar figures were reported in another unit where I had no responsibility. But it was a coping system on my part that became impossible to maintain as the patients being refused admission were clearly suffering from more tractable conditions. There were arguments that the problem of beds was not a clinical problem but rather an administrative or political problem. It was simpler just to fill the unit and hand the problem of beds over to the administrators. Without administrative accountability of some sort, this is simply thrown back as clinical inefficiency in the face of resource shortfalls and does, in fact, mean that the clinician is doing nothing to ensure those who could be treated actually get the treatment they desperately need – he is merely tossing the problem and refusing to meet with his responsibilities.

In any event I found my own particular circumstances becoming quite untenable. Several impassioned altercations with the administration finally led to meetings where I walked out/was thrown out of bad tempered meetings. A formal warning from the administration forced me to seek legal advice to get the record expunged from my service record but it became quite obvious that there were moves afoot to make my place in the system quite unsustainable. At the same time as I approached retirement, it was clear that I would have to do something to improve my own particular circumstances in respect of pension. Thus, in the end, it was easy for me to take early retirement and move elsewhere. It was a decision acceptable to both parties. Perhaps too, my retirement simply allowed the administration to find someone more agreeable to their dictates.

Over the years I also used sabbatical and annual leave to work in other parts of the world. In the Middle East income from oil ensured that each citizen never needed for anything and this included medical care. Again, the technology matched anything on offer anywhere else but because of the open-ended care patients that were regularly transferred to major western centres for little more than a confirmation of the original diagnosis. Brain death as a diagnosis [25] was accepted by the major religion of the region but as is often the case the directives from such authorities did not always permeate down to common practice. The main problem was an insistence beyond an "absolute certainty" in diagnosis. Even in spite of such confirming tests as radioisotope imaging showing no blood flow to the brain, there was a distinct tendency to insist on cessation of heartbeat. Falling foul of such a system always highlighted the notion of time in jail as happened to an elderly South African doctor who faced the accusation that he failed to administer a transfusion to a terminally ill child [26]. As the law in the Middle East seems to be very much of an "eye for an eye" attitude, it is not difficult to understand any reluctance to discuss the subject of cessation of therapy. In essence I found my own particular ethical stance to be at odds with that part of the world.

Following retirement from intensive care, I returned to Ireland to anaesthetic practice in the public service and finally private anaesthesia practice. In Ireland pro-life attitudes are particularly powerful and driven in the recent past by the church and the constitution. According to the constitution, abortion is illegal unless it occurs in order to preserve the life of the mother [27]. In 2013, a new was passed law allowing abortion under certain circumstances. The new law provides for a woman's right to an abortion if her life is at risk, including from suicide. It arose from the unnecessary death of a young mother who developed severe uterine sepsis following spontaneous abortion but was denied an abortion because the foetal heart continued to beat [28]. Someone on the medical/nursing staff is reputed to have remarked that "abortion was impossible because this is a catholic country" [29, 30], The new law, however, was not without strong, if not fanatical protest [31, 32]. In a similar vein euthanasia or assisted suicide is illegal. In spite of this, there is widespread discussion on the topic but anyone attempting to adequately dissect the argument runs the risk of annoying militant pro-life groups prepared to use force to stop such discussion [33]. In fairness, over the 40 years plus of moving backwards and forwards from the country, it has become far more secular allowing previously taboo subjects such as divorce and gay marriage to become law but abortion as a pro-choice event is still far from having legal sanction as is assisted suicide although they are more openly discussed and the *zeitgeist* does appear to be moving in the direction of approval.

All that aside, the main reason for throwing in the towel was more an insidious loss of confidence rather than any assertions of incompetence due to age. Working in private anaesthesia practice, it was seldom possible to undertake a decent medical examination of the patient and decisions to proceed were often taken quickly while falling back on many years of experience in order to deal with a patient. But there was that niggling thought that there was always going to be the statistical outlier who was going to cause problems under anaesthesia with a bad outcome and consequent gimlet eye of the law [3] – like the patient who called me to recovery to tell me he was sorry he did not inform me that his brother had malignant hyperpyrexia even though he had denied this on the admission form! In the end I had just had enough.

Now, I too, face my own demons and have to experience medical practice at the sharp end as a patient. I am still formulating my views on that but have always been troubled by the notion that to deal with a patient to the point that everything has been done to save life and then, when there is no longer any chance of survival, declare that everything has been done and walk away leaving the patient to die alone and abandoned is a particularly noxious form of paternalism. That is nothing more than an emollient to the dictates of society that at one moment demands the autonomous right of the patient to live his life yet denies that same autonomy in the manner of death. But then little has changed since the time of the Epicureans.

References

1. http://www.newyorker.com/magazine/2015/05/18/anatomy-of-error.
2. Dietrich D. The logic of failure: recognising and avoiding error in complex situations. English translation. Metropolitan Books; 1996. ISBN 0-201-47948-6.
3. Keats AS. Anaesthesia mortality in perspective. Anaesth Analg. 1990;71:113–9.
4. Shaw GB. Preferances by George Bernard Shaw. Odhams Press Ltd; 1938.
5. Wright R, Sykes MK. et al. Intermittent positive pressure respiration in tetanus neonatorum. The Lancet. 1961;678.
6. Dwan K, Altman DG, Ionnidas JPA. et al. Systematic review of the empirical evidence of study publication bias and outcome reporting bias. PLoS One. 2008;3(e3081).
7. Miller DR. Publication fraud: implications to the individual and to the speciality. Curr Opin Anaesthesiol. 2011;24:154–9.
8. Bruce G, Charlton MD. The zombie science of evidence-based medicine: a personal retrospective. A commentary on Djulbegovic, B, Guyatt GH. Ashcroft RE. Cancer Control. 2009;16:158–68.
9. Sarwar U, Nicolau M, Fraud and deceit in medical research. J Res Med Sci. 2012;17(11):1077–81. PMCID: PMC3702092.
10. Foster C. Choosing life, choosing death: the tyranny of autonomy in medical ethics and law. Hart Pubishers; 2009. ISBN: 978-1-84113-929-6.
11. vanDellen A. GMC: time to reconsider the civil standard of proof. Ann R Coll Surg Engl. 2013;95(Suppl):XX–XX.
12. The journal, law society of Scotland. http://www.journalonline.co.uk/Magazine/53-9/1005659.aspx#.VVwwB0ZdxiE.
13. Caplan RA. The closed claims project: looking back, looking forward. ASA Newsl. 1999;63(6):7–9.
14. Pirsig RM. Zen and the art of motorcycle maintenance. ISBN 0-553-27747-2.
15. Dorner D. The logic of failure. Metropolitan Books; 1996. ISBN 0-201-47948-6.

16. Deborah T. et al. Medical bankruptcy in the United States, 2007: results of a national study David U. Himmelstein. Am J Med. 2009;122(8):741–46.
17. Murray K. http://www.saturdayeveningpost.com/2013/03/06/in-the-magazine/health-in-the-magazine/how-doctors-die.html.
18. WHO definition of Health: "Health is a state of complete physical, mental and social well-being and not merely the absence of disease or infirmity" Preamble to the Constitution of the World Health Organization as adopted by the International Health Conference, New York, 19–22 June, 1946; signed on 22 July 1946 by the representatives of 61 States (Official Records of the World Health Organization, no. 2, p. 100) and entered into force on 7 April 1948.
19. Hardin G. Tragedy of the commons. Science. 1968;162(3859):1243–8.
20. http://edition.cnn.com/2013/07/18/opinion/mayer-end-of-life-care/.
21. http://edition.cnn.com/2014/01/11/world/meast/obit-ariel-sharon/.
22. http://www.cbsnews.com/news/nelson-mandela-on-life-support/.
23. http://southafrica.shafaqna.com/EN/ZA/222575.
24. Lyons RA, Wareham K. et al. Population requirement for adult critical care beds: a prospective, quantitative and qualitative study. The Lancet. 2000;35:595–8.
25. Islam and brain death: http://www.themodernreligion.com/misc/hh/brain-death.html; http://www.nytimes.com/1999/02/06/world/in-islam-brain-death-ends-life-support.html.
26. http://www.independent.co.uk/news/world/middle-east/south-african-doctor-held-in-uae-jail-on-10yearold-charge-8208039.html.
27. Charleton P, McDermott, PA, Bolger, M. Criminal law. Dublin: Butterworths; 1999. p. 518. ISBN 1854758454.
28. BBC News. Woman dies after abortion request 'refused' at Galway hospital. 14 Nov 2012.
29. Dalby D. Religious remark confirmed in Irish abortion case. The New York Times. 11 Apr 2013.
30. Gynaecology expert to head Savita investigation team. Irish Examiner. 17 Nov 2012. Retrieved 18 Nov 2012.
31. http://www.thejournal.ie/abortion-protest-dublin-repeal-the-8th-1630053-Aug2014/.
32. http://newsbusters.org/blogs/tim-graham/2015/03/13/irelands-pro-lifers-hold-challenging-media-bias-rally-dublin.
33. 2009 euthanasia protesters stop discussion of euthanasia. http://www.fatima.org/news/newsviews/jvnews042309.asp.

Chapter 7
The Aging Intensivist and Academia

Thomas P. Bleck

> *Critical care is a young man's game.*
>
> —*Allan Ropper MD*

Throughout my education and my professional life, I was usually the youngest one around. It came as quite a shock a few years ago, then, when I looked about and discovered that I was one of the oldest full-time neurointensivists in the country, perhaps in the world, and also one of the oldest practicing intensivists of any sort. This realization led me to some consideration of how I arrived in this position and what I should plan to do in the future. However, these concerns are similar to those of most intensivists as they age. Since the focus of this chapter is specifically on academia, I will concentrate predominantly on the interactions of the various parts of the academic medical center with the role of the older intensivist in particular, with some reference to the aging faculty member in general.

In contrast to my usual preparation for writing a chapter, an exhaustive search of the literature revealed very little quantitative information for citation and discussion and only a small amount of qualitative description. What follows is predominantly personal observation, which experience teaches is potentially faulty and certainly biased; nevertheless, I hope it proves useful to the reader.

I would be remiss in telling this story if I did not give credit to some of my role models and mentors [1] in this journey. John Hubbard ran an undergraduate physiology course at Northwestern that completely redirected my career path from psychology to physiology and thence to medicine. Stuart Levin taught me to be a physician and awakened my interest in infectious diseases. Harold Klawans taught me to be a neurologist and a bedside teacher. Frank Morrell developed my skills as an epileptologist and taught me to think scientifically. Donna Bergen honed my skills as an electroencephalographer. Roger Bone told me that "by constitution you are an intensivist, and you should just admit this and get on with your life"; this simple statement changed my career and with it my life. Fred Wooten taught me to

T.P. Bleck, MD, MCCM, FNCS
Professor of Neurological Sciences, Rush Medical College, Chicago, IL, USA

Director of Clinical Neurophysiology, Rush University Medical Center, Chicago, IL, USA
e-mail: tbleck@gmail.com

© Springer International Publishing Switzerland 2016
D. Crippen (ed.), *The Intensivist's Challenge: Aging and Career Growth in a High-Stress Medical Specialty*, DOI 10.1007/978-3-319-30454-0_7

find and develop talented students, trainees, and junior faculty. David Ansell showed me how to guide colleagues to do better, sometimes against their own impulses.

And then there is Fred Dreifuss, who figures below.

Critical Care Practice in the Academic Environment

Whether in academic or private practice, being an intensivist is physically demanding. However, the academic intensivist is usually surrounded by younger colleagues, particularly residents and fellows, that cushion one from some of the larger physical challenges, such as trying to perform high-quality CPR for more than a few minutes. It is difficult to accept the concept that I no longer have the stamina that I had in the past to handle service in the ICU for a week or two with its attendant long hours and pressures. For me, the first thing that I and others noticed is that I no longer functioned as well as I thought I formerly did in the setting of lack of adequate sleep. The weeks on service with frequent night telephone calls and occasional drives back to the hospital also began to affect my health. My associates noted a problem and for the last few years have arranged for one of the other intensivists to handle these night telephone calls. Over the past few years, I have had progressively less ICU service, replaced by more time interpreting ICU EEG monitoring and helping the other intensivists manage patients with difficult seizure disorders. At the same time, as an institution, we decided to have an adult intensivist present in the hospital at night, which has essentially eliminated the need for intensivists on each service to return to the hospital at night. These accommodations are probably much easier to make in an academic environment than they would be in a practice, where I would probably have had to shift to an outpatient practice for which I am no longer well suited. While I recognize that these changes are beneficial for my health, I miss the day-to-day involvement with the ICU.

Maintaining technical competence as one ages is a concern for all physicians in procedural specialties, but it is a special issue for academic intensivists who must be primarily concerned with teaching and supervising procedures rather than perform-ing them personally. As the size of the critical care team has grown, the opportuni-ties for me to "help out" by placing lines and doing other procedures myself have decreased considerably. In my early days in the neurointensive care unit at the University of Virginia, the medical staff consisted of one attending and two residents taking every-other-night call, so I got to do plenty of procedures myself. As some-one who was accused later in his career of "stealing" such procedures from his trainees, I confess that my fingers still itch when I supervise residents and fellows, but I am now able to restrain myself from jumping in too early. I still relish the request to scrub in and help out when things are difficult, but I realize that the time will come when my skills and physical abilities are no longer equal to the task. Perhaps one of the advantages of the training environment is the constant presence of younger colleagues and trainees who will be quite aware of any decline in intel-lectual or technical performance. It is incumbent on all of us to be certain that they are able to keep our patients safe by pointing out any decrement in abilities.

Teaching

One might assume that a transition from clinical work in the ICU to more teaching time as one ages is a logical transition, but since most of the teaching on a critical care service is done at the bedside, less service means fewer opportunities for teaching at a stage in one's career when one has the most experience to impart.

Teaching is the area of our profession in which I feel most out of step with modern trends. With a long career of varied experiences in critical care, I envision that I have a lot to teach my students, trainees, and younger colleagues; isn't this central to the role of the academic physician? However, medical education has changed tremendously during the course of my career, not entirely negatively, but not so positively either. Clinicians now play a minimal part in the "preclinical" years of medical school, and to the extent that they are involved, it is typically in the teaching of physical diagnosis. I currently have 1 h of contact with first year medical students. The trend toward introducing a longitudinal patient care experience is by definition focused on outpatient physicians, leaving no place for intensivists without office practices.

When students arrive in the intensive care unit in their clerkship years, they have absorbed the unfortunate notion that they will learn by seeing some "interesting" patients, going to lectures, and perhaps reading a little bit. We are teaching them something about diseases, but we are not teaching them to be doctors in this "overt" curriculum. Fortunately for the future of our profession, some of them still want to spend time with their patients and seek out experienced clinicians to begin the process of learning to care for patients and their families. The term "hidden curriculum" usually refers to things students learn from bad examples, but there is also the possibility of a positive hidden curriculum for students who recognize what being a doctor is about.

Teaching residents is even more challenging because of the current work hour rules. As a resident, one needs to take ownership of the patient's problems, but this concept has been replaced by shift work. The most pernicious aspect of the work hour limits is the unsubtle transfer of responsibility for both the continuity of knowledge about the patient and for decision-making from the resident to the attending intensivist. To date, the modest research published about the effects of these changes has not uncovered an advantage to either the patients or the residents. However, it is clear to me that the residents finish this phase of their training with less knowledge, less skill, and less capacity to manage patients independently than did their counterparts who trained two decades earlier. The frequency of handoffs from one team to the next ensures that no one except the attending intensivist has any concept of what should be done. In this environment, the residents do not make enough decisions to understand their consequences and therefore cannot learn to trust (or when appropriate, question) their judgment.

Perhaps the most destructive effect of degrading the residency experience this way is the notion that one can see "enough" of a particular type of patient. I applaud the recording of patients and procedures to help ensure that the resident has sufficiently broad experience, but this should not have been at the expense of the depth of that experience. After over 30 years as an attending intensivist, I have yet to conclude an ICU rotation without seeing something new or gaining experience with a new drug or procedure.

If it were simply a case of me having a less enjoyable teaching experience, I would gladly trade that for some benefit accruing to the patients or the residents. However, no benefits have been demonstrated. I wish I knew how to rectify these problems. At the least, residencies need to be extended for more patient contact.

Research

As an academic, I have been involved in bedside clinical research and large clinical trials throughout my career. An advantage conferred by decades spent developing networks among researchers and publishing in the field is that I am still asked to participate in national and international trials as an executive committee member, as a safety monitor, or as a member of the data safety and monitoring committee. This allows me to remain on the cutting edge of clinical research.

A commonly cited truism is that scientists in various fields make their most important contributions at different ages. Physicists were thought to reach their peaks in their 20s, chemists in their 30s, and biologists and physicians in their 40s. While it is not clear that this was ever really correct, and in my lifetime of observation I have many examples of later-blooming investigators, there is a sense that the general concept of research productivity waning with age is correct. (However, a recent analysis contends that in the past few decades, this diminution with advancing years is no longer so prominent, especially in medicine [2].)

There is a considerable literature about the development of research productivity and the acquisition of external financial support among early career physician scientists [3], but not much is written about research activities as they approach the later portions of their careers. At some point, we each decide that there is no reason to prepare another research proposal or grant application personally, but rather that one should focus on helping younger colleagues develop their skills in constructing a competitive application.

For the last few years, my major research efforts have been devoted to serving as a mentor for the early career grants of junior investigators and to service on data safety and monitoring boards. These activities have allowed me to help guide clinical research and to remain part of the cutting edge.

Administration

Spending more time and effort on administration seems like a natural way to make use of accumulated experience. I served for several years as the associate chief medical officer for critical care, a position for which both I and my superiors thought

I was well suited. This position allowed me to devote thought and time to some major projects, such as the design and construction of a new hospital tower which now houses almost all of the institution's intensive care units, as well as the emergency department.

One should be careful, however, about assuming purely administrative positions without some direct patient care involvement. It is too often the case that this leads to loss of connection with the purpose of our work.

National and International Teaching and Society Involvement

It is hopefully apparent from the list of fellowships (and one mastership) after my name at the start of this chapter that I am a joiner. These and other organizations have been at the core of my professional development. Some of my mentors were also joiners, while others were only minimally involved in academic medicine outside of their own institutions. While there is no single path through academic life, these organizations have been very important to me, and while I am encouraged by the vigor with which my younger colleagues have continued to build and strengthen them, the fact that I am no longer in leadership positions within them is a sign of aging that I struggle to accept gracefully.

I began attending national scientific meetings as a resident and realized that the world outside of my own institution has a lot to teach me. I also wanted to participate in this world, so I began submitting abstracts and joining interesting committees. At the conclusion of one such committee meeting in 1988, I asked one of my friends, Dan Hanley, where he was going next; he replied that a small group of neurologists interested in critical care were getting together to request some platform time for neurocritical care abstracts at the next American Academy of Neurology annual meeting. Already having heard Roger Bone's assessment, I became part of that group, which led to considerable involvement in numerous AAN committees and sections over the rest of my career. Roger also got me involved in the Society of Critical Care Medicine, which has been central to my professional evolution; I invested 12 years on the SCCM council, which helped me immeasurably, and I believe has helped both neurocritical care and general critical care as well. Now that my terms on the council have concluded, however, I feel disconnected from the direction of the SCCM; I suppose this is natural as younger members take on the mantle of leadership, but this transition was the first time at which I recognized that the passage of years was going to close some doors for me. In recent years, I have been as likely to be called upon to contribute to guidelines [4] as I am to help design or conduct original research. I hope this is a sign of wisdom and experience.

In the late 1990s, there was enough of a critical mass of neurointensivists to consider the possibility of a society devoted to neurocritical care [5]. I was not conscious of this aspect at that time, but I had suddenly moved from being the young buck to being the senior wise man. By 2002, we had drafted a set of bylaws for what is now the Neurocritical Care Society, and I was elected the founding president. This society has clearly been the high point of my professional career. As a past president, I remain more connected to the operations of the NCS than I am with the other organizations of which I am a member.

Fritz (Fred) Dreifuss was, in my view, the leading epileptologist of his era. Early in our friendship, he explained to me that when he began his work in epilepsy care and research, the field was seen as unrewarding to a neurologist beyond the study of the Jacksonian march. He decided that he would put epilepsy on the map for neurology, medicine, and patient care in general. Part of his strategy for doing so was to accept every offer to speak about epilepsy, regardless of the size of the venue and the difficulties of traveling to it. I could see that this strategy had been successful in its own right and that by raising worldwide interest, he had contributed not only with his own research, but had spurred others to make the tremendous advances in medical therapy, epilepsy surgery, and the psychological and social care of patients that we now take almost for granted. I decided that I would follow a similar strategy to help move neurocritical care from the cottage industry that it was in 1990 to the vibrant and essential part of medicine that it is today. The reader can decide whether he or she agrees with this assessment. I treated invitations to write chapters and editorials the same way; these were (and remain) vehicles to make people aware that the patients of neurointensivists can benefit tremendously from our current work and that at the same time so much remains to be accomplished.

As the field has grown, however, there are an increasing number of outstanding researchers and speakers who can fill this role. I am still pleased to be invited to speak, but I realize that some of my appeal is more historical than cutting edge, no matter how up-to-date I may strive to be. While I recognize this as a natural progression, I still find it disconcerting.

End-of-Career Planning

The analogy to end-of-life planning is intentional. Several years ago I accepted a position as a department chair, in which my major focus shifted from my own work to the professional and personal development of students, trainees, and especially junior faculty members. Subsequently, I was offered the opportunity to plan and orchestrate the move of critical care services from an aging physical plant into a new facility. Each step in this process has been a move forward, but I have now come to realize that there are not going to be that many opportunities for further motion.

Many of us have seen mentors and colleagues whose faculties begin to fail before they feel ready to retire. This statement is typically followed by one indicating that the author hopes that his or her colleagues will let them know that the time has come for them to step away from any activities that could lead to less-than-optimal patient outcomes or from teaching that is not current or is patently wrong. While this is true, I hope that I will be able to recognize such problems in myself before anyone else does and move myself out of the way while people still view me as a star in my game, even if I am no longer at the top of it.

I think it is incumbent on those of us facing this problem to help design systems to identify declining performance and to either treat problems that are remediable or move colleagues out of harm's way when the problems cannot be managed. This concern is visible in the popular press as well as the medical literature [6]. While there has been some work in this area [7], much remains to be done, and there is no one better positioned to take responsibility for it than we are. If we are still competent, excited by the work, and learning, we are not ready to retire.

Perhaps, as my wife says, I should cut back to full-time.

> *Though wise men at their end know dark is right,*
> *Because their words had forked no lightning they*
> *Do not go gentle into that good night.*
> —Dylan Thomas

Acknowledgement I am indebted to my wife, Laura Friedland, for a critical review of the manuscript and several important suggestions.

References

1. Mentor was the tutor of Telemachus, the son of Odysseus and Penelope, in Homer's Odyssey. Mentor is a proper noun, not a verb.
2. Jones BF, Weinberg BA. Age dynamics in scientific creativity. Proc Natl Acad Sci U S A. 2011;108:18910–4.
3. Garrison HH, Deschamps AM. NIH research funding and early career physician scientists: continuing challenges in the 21st century. FASEB J. 2014;28:1049–58.
4. Kotloff RM, Blosser S, Fulda GJ, et al. Management of the Potential Organ Donor in the ICU: Society of Critical Care Medicine/American College of Chest Physicians/Association of Organ Procurement Organizations Consensus Statement. Crit Care Med. 2015;43:1291–325.
5. Korbakis G, Bleck TP. The evolution of neurocritical care. Crit Care Clin. 2014;30:657–71.
6. Tarkan L. As doctors age, worries about their ability grow. NY Times. 24 Jan 2011.
7. Durning SJ, Arino AR, Holmboe E, et al. Aging and cognitive performance: challenges and implications for physicians practicing in the 21st century. J Cont Educ Health Prof. 2010;30:153–60.

Chapter 8
The Critical Care Physician and a Career in Industry: Reflections and Recommendations

Donald B. Chalfin

Introduction

Physicians often consider career changes after years in clinical and academic practice for many reasons, including a desire to embrace new challenges, a need to physically and intellectually "recharge," and a wish to "redirect" one's energies and talents. Private industry offers many opportunities for the well-seasoned and experienced clinician, and physicians increasingly have assumed vital and indispensible roles in pharmaceutical, device, and diagnostic companies, with many physician often assuming key leadership and management positions. The role of physicians in industry has significantly expanded and become more diverse largely due to the advances in medical science and healthcare delivery along with the increased complexities associated with clinical medicine, research, and development and the multifaceted challenges associated with bringing a product to market. A career in industry can be personally exciting and professionally fulfilling for the mid-career physician; however, anyone who contemplates such a move should understand the skills, temperament, and mindset required to thrive and succeed. This chapter will provide a brief overview of my perspective of some of the key aspects that the physician who is considering a mid-career change into industry needs to consider prior to making a move.

Industry: Basic Definitions and Focus

In the colloquial sense, most individuals tend to think of industry as a "catch-all" phase synonymous with the big pharmaceutical companies, especially the large, diversified multinational drug corporations. While the traditional multinational drug

D.B. Chalfin, MD, MS, MPH, FCCP, FCCM
Jefferson College of Population Health of Thomas Jefferson University, Philadelphia, PA, USA
e-mail: dbchalfin@gmail.com

© Springer International Publishing Switzerland 2016
D. Crippen (ed.), *The Intensivist's Challenge: Aging and Career Growth in a High-Stress Medical Specialty*, DOI 10.1007/978-3-319-30454-0_8

companies certainly account for a large share of the industry sector in terms of people employed, research and development (R&D), and market share, industry is much broader than "Big Pharma," for it includes small, mid-size, and large companies dedicated not only to drugs but vaccines, diagnostics, and medical devices. It also goes beyond this scope and also includes companies that focus on services versus research and development and product manufacturing and distribution. These service companies include insurers and payers, contract research organizations (CROs), management consulting firms, health economics and outcomes research companies, and marketing and market research organizations. In addition, biotechnology has also changed the face of industry, and thus, companies and industry can be further conceptualized into the more traditional organizations dedicated to "small molecules" and conventional healthcare products versus many of the newer corporations that focus dedicated to biotechnology-related disciplines, including gene expression technology, genomics, proteomics, medical informatics, and personalized medicine. For the purposes of this article, the term 'industry' will refer to those organizations dedicated to pharmaceuticals, diagnostic tests, medical devices, vaccines, and related products, compounds, and agents.

Reality Check: Dispelling Common Myths

Many perceptions abound as to what the physician should expect and anticipate with a career in industry. At the outset, one must dispense with the commonly held belief that a job in industry is a transition to retirement. While industry positions do not have the clinical stresses associated with the life of an intensivist or other physicians, including the physical challenges and emotional demands of night, weekend, and holiday duty, or the pressure, tension, and uncertainty associated with the care of the critically ill and injured, industry jobs nevertheless present its own set of pressures and challenges and often demand long hours, frequent, and distant travel that often last for extended periods; the ability to manage multiple projects, tasks, and teams; and the often unending stresses associated with adhering to a timeline and meeting vital corporate goals that often have great influence with respect to a drug's, a product's, or even a company's success.

On top of this, those who opt to move into industry should quickly shed the notion that one's education, training, and experience as a physician are all that one needs in order to succeed and advance. Clearly, the physician's perspective is vital and indispensible in almost all phases of product discovery, development, and commercialization, as physicians via their direct experience in dealing with patients are often the only ones who can best articulate and advocate for, to use the business vernacular, the needs of the intended "client" [1]. However, product development and delivery, at all stages, is a costly, time-consuming, multifunctional, and resource-intensive endeavor that requires the contributions from multiple disciplines of many experts, ranging from basic scientists, engineers, mathematicians, chemists, biologists, database professionals, and computer scientists to biostatisticians, systems analysts, clinical trial professionals, pharmacologists, manufacturing, and quality control experts to financial managers, sales, marketing, and commercial experts to regulatory specialists, safety scientists, pharmacovigilance specialists, and legal counselors. Drug and product development may even require the efforts and contributions of multiple companies and organizations, including collaborations between industry, government, healthcare organizations, and academia [2]. As Love writes in a piece referring to drug discovery and development, "It takes much more talent and experience than one individual can master to file a successful new drug application, design a robust clinical development program, and file a new drug application" [3]. On top of this, drug and product development has a prolonged and protracted timeline. The path from "molecule to market" can take many years and paths, and thus, physicians accustomed to the immediate returns and rewards associated with patient care will need to reorient themselves to the long-term perspective and the different reward system associated with most projects, tasks, and initiatives.

There is also a perception, perhaps fueled by the changes in healthcare financing and delivery, that an industry position provides a reasonable level of stability in terms of employment guarantees and job security. While this belief may have been the norm in years past when individuals in healthcare and other industries could count upon steady job advancement and dependable employee-employer commitment and often held jobs for many years and even for several decades, one is more likely to encounter flux and frequent change. In fact, uncertainly has probably become than the standard in industry, due to such factors as marketplace uncertainty, corporate mergers and acquisitions, product obsolescence and technology shifts, changes in medical reimbursement, product coverage, and healthcare delivery, and the general globalization of the world economy.

Large Versus Small

Job security is implicitly linked to a company's stability, and thus, the likelihood for its sustained growth and its overall financial health is frequently linked to its on-market portfolio and product pipeline. However, stability, performance, and scope also depend upon a company's market capitalization with respect to publically held companies and the stage and level of financial development with respect to privately held corporations. With respect to the latter, physicians and others are increasingly recruited and employed by smaller start-up companies. Start-up organizations appeal to many because they offer the challenge of being part of the formative stage of an organization at the "ground floor" that may have vast potential significant medical impact and large financial payoffs down the road. Thus, for an individual willing to take on the inherent risk associated with working for a new and smaller venture, often in an untraditional and less-hierarchical organization, a start-up company may represent the right environment and opportunity. One just needs to reckon with the fact that start-up companies, especially those in the earlier and often formative stages, tend to have a small portfolio of products or drugs in development and may be years from regulatory approval and entering the market. They are frequently dependent upon the ability to raise money from venture capitalists and other investors over a prolonged period of time and hence require a willingness to deal with such factors – especially at the outset – as minimal benefits, lower and occasionally uncertain remuneration, and long hours at work engaged in tasks and activities that are traditionally performed by teams of dedicated individuals in larger, more established corporations.

Physician's Roles and Responsibilities Within Industry

Regardless of company size, financing, or focus, positions for physicians in industry generally have a common structure in terms of responsibilities, titles, and hierarchy. Physician's responsibilities are often quite variable and depend upon the company's product line, portfolio, and pipeline and its overall area of scientific emphasis and expertise. However, most physician's responsibilities and jobs are generally reduced to two main areas of concentration: clinical development and medical affairs. Clinical development generally refers to the design and development of research trials throughout most of the stages of the product lifecycle. This includes, to use the paradigm of drug development, the preclinical stage, early-stage development that captures Phase I and Phase II studies, and the later-stage research studies of Phase III (and occasionally Phase IIB) and the large, multicenter, often multinational pivotal clinical trials that are performed for regulatory approval. A physician's role and the projects and initiatives that one will work on will largely be determined by his or her expertise, not just in terms of clinical training and specialty certification but also one's experience in research methods, clinical trial development, study management, laboratory investigation, data analysis and interpretation, publication, and translational research.

Medical affairs activities include, among other tasks and responsibilities, varying degrees of clinical research with the focus largely upon Phase IV and to a lesser extent Phase III. Physicians in medical affairs also have more contact with their commercial and regulatory colleagues and also tend to have responsibilities related to a broader range of activities, including outcomes research, health economics, medical education, publication planning, risk management, patient safety, and pharmacovigilance; the development and supervision of patient registries; field and customer support; medical liaison activities; and the organization of physician panels, advisory boards, and other related assemblies. Despite this dichotomy between clinical development and medical affairs, there is frequently significant overlap between the two, not only in terms of content and collaboration but also in terms of how responsibilities are delineated and how positions, departments, and teams are defined.

From the standpoint of job hierarchy and titles, most corporations employ the same general framework in terms of managerial responsibilities, seniority, compensation, and organizational position. Physicians starting out in industry, especially those fresh out of training usually begin as an associate medical director. More senior physicians, however, may begin as a medical director or even higher, depending upon their experience, level of board certification, research productivity and publication history, administrative experience, and prior history with industry. An associate medical director often has few, if any, direct reports, usually concentrate on just one or two projects and initiatives, and largely focuses on tactical versus strategic activities. Medical directors often have one or more direct reports, have broader responsibilities in terms of project scope, and tend to assume increasing levels of strategic responsibilities that may involve more cross-divisional functions and long-range planning. In most organizations, the next tier includes the senior and executive medical directors, followed by vice-president and then chief medical officer positions. As one would surmise, each level is usually associated with increasing managerial and strategic responsibilities, more direct reports, and a greater role in senior management and leadership teams with more cross-divisional and – depending upon the corporate size and structure – cross-organizational interactions.

Compensation

Industry compensation depends upon several factors, including corporate size and structure (e.g., privately held versus public), years of experience, and specific position (e.g., director, senior director, etc.). In general, remuneration is derived from several sources, including salary, bonuses and incentives (which are usually linked to some combination of individual, group, divisional, and overall corporate performance), stock options and grants, and other employee-related benefits, from health insurance to retirement funds. Physicians and others who are employed by large public companies usually earn a steady salary along with associated annual increases, and most have related income (i.e., bonuses) that are related to their position, their level of responsibility and seniority, and other organizational aspects. Furthermore, physicians and employees in many companies, especially the larger, publically held organizations, are often provided with stock grants and/ or options.

Compensation in smaller companies, especially start-ups, is usually competitive but may be less, depending upon the stage of development and financing. However, physicians and other employees – especially those in key leadership and managerial positions, often receive a significant level of stock, usually in the form of options that have the potential for a significant payout in the future. While specific levels of compensation are beyond the scope of this chapter, physicians can generally expect to be well compensated with relatively competitive salaries, albeit with a higher level of uncertainty relative to academic and institutional clinical practice [2].

Other Considerations

Certain clinical specialties and disciplines, such as cardiology, oncology, molecular biology, infectious diseases, clinical pharmacology, and immunology, are likely to have more opportunities than others in industry due to the fact that they represent areas of active research, development, and commercialization or cover disciplines that have common need across various industries; critical care physicians have many unique skills that make them very desirable in the industry world. Critical care by its very nature requires expertise in multiple clinical and medical disciplines, and as such, the intensivist can easily work and adapt to many different content areas in industry. Furthermore, critical care by its very nature is team oriented, and thus, critical care physicians are used to working collaboratively in large, multifunctional, multidisciplinary teams, a skill that will serve one extremely well in the industry setting. Lastly, critical care physicians are likely to be detail oriented and have the ability to "multitask," another skill that will be required in most industry positions.

Despite my belief that critical care provides an excellent foundation for a successful and fulfilling career in industry, one nevertheless has to appreciate that physicians frequently lack key abilities that are helpful and even necessary to succeed and contribute, and thus, physicians who go into industry must be amenable to learning new skills and embracing new challenges distinct from clinical and academic medicine. The physician, as previously stated, serves as the voice of the patient and as the key clinical expert, and as such, he or she must draw upon and even leverage his or her medical knowledge. To this end, physicians in industry must maintain their clinical competency, and I would even suggest that they continue to maintain a clinical edge with some level of patient care activity, something which many companies support and even encourage. Yet it is probably safe to posit that physicians often lack business and management training and experience, and unless they have had prior experience or have earned additional degrees or certificates, one would be well advised to acquire expertise in or at least exposure key business, management, and analytical activities such as project management, financial and quantitative methods, and database analysis and interpretation. In addition, while most physicians are used to presenting and communicating medical and scientific ideas to their colleagues, the ability to present key medical concepts and facts, such as findings from clinical trials or general information about clinical medicine and disease processes, requires experience and exposure. From a managerial standpoint, many physicians who move into industry may not be used to direct supervision of others outside of the medical, nursing, or clinical realm, and thus, a physician who has direct reports should consider internal and external support to ease his or her transition. Lastly, physicians need to learn how to develop and detail concrete goals, as almost all corporations require clearly defined specific goal setting that describes objectives, tasks, and even timelines that are specific, clearly defined, and measurable.

Concluding Thoughts

Industry represents a viable and frequently an exciting option for the experienced physician who seeks a career change and also wants to actively embrace new challenges in a different environment. It is important to reiterate that industry should not be viewed as a retirement option or pathway as almost all jobs demand complete dedication and commitment. As with any important career choice, those who consider moving to industry should carefully consider all options and weigh the benefits and shortcomings. From my perspective and experience, despite the need to acquire new skills and reorient one's overall focus from the individual patient to a broader, population approach and a longer time horizon, one of the greatest rewards in industry, given the right opportunity, organization, and "fit," is the chance to use one's training and experience to advance clinical practice and medical care from a different perspective.

References

1. Timpane J. Everywhere and then some: physicians making careers in biopharmaceuticals. JAMA. 1998;279:1401.
2. Leppert D. Glanzman: on being a neurologist in industry. Ann Neurol. 2013;73:319–26.
3. Love TW. Transition from academia to industry: a personal account. Exp Biol Med. 2006;231(11):1682–4.

Chapter 9
Race and the ICU

Errington C. Thompson

I'm standing in line at a relatively crowded local restaurant. My stethoscope is around my neck because, like my wedding ring, it seems I never take it off. I also have my ID badge from the hospital clipped on to my blue blazer. A short middle-aged man yells from across the restaurant, "Mr. Thompson!" Almost nobody calls me Mr. Thompson. Friends will call me, "Errington" and others will call me, "Dr. Thompson." I reply, "Yes?" The man walks over to me as he says, "Did you go to State?" "I grew up in Dallas and went to college at Emory University in Atlanta." A real curious look came across this man's face. He was initially sure that I was someone he used to know now he isn't so sure.

Mistaken identity is not unusual. It happens. It happens more often when a person of one race is trying to identify a person of another race [1]. When I wore a white medical jacket in the hospital, it was relatively common for someone to say, "Hi Dr. So-and-So." Dr. So-and-So is a black physician and I am also a black physician. It isn't that we look the same. We do not. I am relatively tall at 6' 2" and Dr. So-and-So is short and stocky. For the most part, I would like to think that these people are trying to be friendly but don't take the time to really focus on facial features.

In 2002, the Institute of Medicine released *Unequal Treatment* [2]. This was a critical indictment of the medical community with regard to race and ethnic disparities. There were several critical findings:

- *Finding 1–1*: Racial and ethnic disparities in healthcare exist and, because they are associated with worse outcomes in many cases, are unacceptable.
- *Finding 2–1*: Racial and ethnic disparities in healthcare occur in the context of broader historic and contemporary social and economic inequality and evidence of persistent racial and ethnic discrimination in many sectors of American life.

E.C. Thompson, MD
Department of Surgery, Marshall University,
1600 Medical Center Dr, Suite 2500, Huntington, WV 25705, USA
e-mail: thompsoner@marshall.edu; erringtonthompson@gmail.com

© Springer International Publishing Switzerland 2016
D. Crippen (ed.), *The Intensivist's Challenge: Aging and Career Growth in a High-Stress Medical Specialty*, DOI 10.1007/978-3-319-30454-0_9

- *Finding 3–1*: Many sources – including health systems, healthcare providers, patients, and utilization managers – may contribute to racial and ethnic disparities in healthcare.
- *Finding 4–1*: Bias, stereotyping, prejudice, and clinical uncertainty on the part of healthcare providers may contribute to racial and ethnic disparities in healthcare. While indirect evidence from several lines of research supports this statement, a greater understanding of the prevalence and influence of these processes is needed and should be sought through research.
- *Finding 4–2*: A small number of studies suggest that racial and ethnic minority patients are more likely than white patients to refuse treatment. These studies find that differences in refusal rates are generally small and that minority patient refusal does not fully explain healthcare disparities.

Several years ago, I was sitting in an ethics committee meeting. We were receiving a lecture on healthcare disparities. One of my colleagues raised his hand to ask why we were listening to this lecture. He stated clearly that he had never discriminated against a patient nor anyone else in his life. He actually said that this lecture was a waste of his time.

Now, I am not sure if my colleague was being facetious or not. He seemed to be serious. Race and ethnicity are touchy subjects in American society. Nobody wants to be called a racist. Nobody wants to be labeled as a physician, healthcare provider who discriminates against certain types of patients. Unfortunately, we all have prejudices [3].

There is a theory in the field of anthropology that supposes prejudice may actually have a survival advantage. When we were living in small clans, it was critically important for us to be able to recognize the members of our clan. Think about it. If a stranger comes up to your group, more bad things can happen than good things. A stranger can take your food. A stranger can take your women. A stranger can injure or murder your men. All of these bad things can be avoided by recognizing strangers and avoiding them. On the other hand, clans are excellent at spreading tradition. In a small clique, you can tell your cousins, your offspring, and your neighbors to avoid hazards and embrace certain practices which have been successful [4]. Whether prejudice has a survival advantage or not, it is clear that we all have prejudices. Whether we are prejudiced when it comes to race or hair color or obesity or whatever, we do have prejudices and those prejudices can color our judgment.

The trauma literature has tons of articles which correlate the severity of injury to mortality. The Injury Severity Score [5], which has been used for years, basically takes injuries and scores them. The higher the injury severity score, the higher the likelihood of death. Yet, Cornwell et al. investigated the National Trauma Databank, and their results were published in 2008 [6]. The authors looked at insurance status, race, and injury severity. They analyzed over 370,000 patients. The mortality rate for whites was 5.7 %. The mortality rate for blacks was 8.2 %. The mortality rate for Hispanics was 9.1 %. When whites were compared to blacks or Hispanics, they had a statistically significant lower mortality rate. The mortality rate was almost twice for uninsured patients versus insured patients (4.4 % and 8.6 %). This was statistically significant ($p < 0.005$). Even when the authors adjusted for injury severity, blacks and Hispanics with insurance had a higher mortality rate than did white patients with insurance. This data clearly suggests that insurance status and race play a very important role in mortality. Here's the crazy thing about this data. Most trauma surgeons would argue that trauma is one of the most protocolized fields in medicine. From the moment that they enter the trauma system in the field, patients are being placed in one protocol or another. If the patient is hypotensive and a victim of blunt trauma, we have one protocol. If the patient is normotensive with penetrating trauma, they are in a different protocol. How can patients who are being taken care in extensively researched evidence-based protocols have racial disparities?

Over the last 20 years, protocols have sprung up in the ICU. The Surviving Sepsis Campaign is one such protocol. This protocol is fairly simple and is supported by the Society of Critical Care Medicine and the Centers for Disease Control [7, 8]. The basic tenets of the protocol are to recognize sepsis early, give patient appropriate antibiotics early in their disease process, and to adequately resuscitate the patient early and aggressively. Again, much like in the trauma population, there really should not be any healthcare disparities in patients with sepsis.

A.M. Esper and colleagues investigated patients who were entered into the National Hospital Discharge Survey from 1979 through 2003 (the majority of these patients probably were not included in any nationwide sepsis protocol) [9]. There were over 12 million reported cases of sepsis during the 25-year study timeframe. The main hospital length of stay for sepsis was higher for blacks than for whites. The incidence of organ dysfunction was also higher for blacks than for whites. Interestingly, case fatality rates were similar between the two groups.

In the *Journal of Critical Care Medicine*, Dombrovskly et al. studied all patients with a diagnosis of sepsis in New Jersey in 2002 [10]. Although their data set was significantly smaller than Esper's, they still identified over 24,000 patients who were admitted with a diagnosis of sepsis. The authors found the relative risk of sepsis in black patients was greater than that of white patients. There was a difference in the relative risk in different age categories, but the risk remained larger for blacks than whites for all age groups. The age-adjusted fatality rates for blacks and whites were not statistically different. Curiously, blacks were more likely than whites to be admitted to the hospital or the ICU from the emergency room with a diagnosis of sepsis. The length of stay both in the hospital and in the ICU was greater for blacks than for whites.

Exactly what are we trying to do with this data anyway? With most investigations, the researchers are trying to improve outcomes. Are we really trying to improve outcomes for a specific minority group? Are we really trying to improve care for blacks and Hispanics alone? By studying these discrepancies, can we improve care for all patients? My somewhat sheepish answer is, "I do not know." If, on the other hand, our goal is to simply point out that these discrepancies exist, I am not sure that publishing more data on racial and ethnic disparities is worth the time and the effort of the investigators.

One of the biggest problems with studying racial discrepancies is trying to figure out what the definitions are. In critical care, we have struggled with definitions of respiratory failure, multiple organ dysfunction syndrome, and adult respiratory distress syndrome. After a robust debate in the literature, there is usually a conference in which the definitions are hammered out among experts. In the United States, race is somewhat nebulous [11]. As far as I know, no conference of experts on this topic has been convened. There has been no universally agreed-upon definition. It is kind of like the definition that Supreme Court Justice Potter Stewart used for obscenity [12]. He said he could not define it, but he recognized it when he saw it. Describing a black man, an Asian woman, or a Hispanic child eludes a specific definition, but, at least in the United States, we all have a picture instantly of what this person looks like in our minds.

The fact that the majority of the literature on race relations and racial discrepancies depends upon self-described racial classification diminishes its accuracy. Most of us have heard the story of former NAACP employee Rachel Dolezal [13]. Basically, both of Rachel's parents are white. Over the years, she changed her appearance and began to identify herself as black. Although cases like these are rare, we know the opposite is true. Light-skinned blacks and Hispanics have long been identified as white. What percentage of blacks, whites, and Hispanics has changed their racial categorization? We do not have the answer to this question.

Although this literature is confusing and the different races are hard to define, I do think that there is some validity in studying racial discrepancies. First of all, we must improve healthcare for all of the patients that we serve. If studying racial discrepancies helps improve outcomes, then we need to vigorously investigate their root causes. Secondly, we need to be able to bring individualized healthcare to the bedside. We need to begin treating patients as they would like to be treated. If that means that we need to learn to be more culturally aware of our patients' needs, then that is the direction that medicine needs to follow.

End-of-life issues is one area of critical care in which blacks and Hispanics really differ from their white counterparts [14]. Nursing home residents, in one study, were less likely to fill out do not resuscitate orders, living wills, and other end-of-life orders if they were black or Hispanic. Blacks and Hispanics were more likely to want aggressive treatment at the end of life. These findings were followed up by another study showing that blacks are more likely to want feeding tubes in spite of having a terminal illness. Black patients claimed that they would want more aggressive intervention than their white counterparts, if they were to find themselves in a permanently unconscious state. Studying these types of differences among whites, blacks, Hispanics, and other racial minorities is integral to our doing our jobs as critical care physicians. We do not want to assume what kind of care a patient would want. We need to be empathetic with our patients and listen carefully to their surrogates. We need to work hard to avoid injecting our own bias into these end-of-life discussions.

One study showed that blacks perceived the role of their family members as protecting them from the healthcare system [15]. If this is true, then it means that we are failing as healthcare providers. We need to do whatever we can to empower families and patients. They must feel that they are in control of their healthcare or we are not doing our jobs. Our goal must be to deliver the healthcare that patients want and deserve as opposed to the healthcare that we think they need. The distinction is subtle, but important.

In the local restaurant, the portly white man walks up to me and shakes my hand. It is now clear to him that I'm not his friend. We exchange pleasantries. He shares with me that he and his friend had some great times in college playing music into the early morning hours.

Racial disparities exist throughout healthcare. As healthcare providers, we need to develop strategies in order to combat the effects of these disparities on our patients and improve outcomes. We need to develop an environment in which our patients (of all races) feel that they are empowered and in control of their own healthcare.

References

1. Rutledge JP. They all look alike: the inaccuracy of cross-racial identifications. Am J Crim Law. Spring 2001:211–4.
2. Nelson AR, Smedley BD, Stith AY. Unequal treatment: confronting racial and ethnic disparities in health care. Washington DC: National Academies Press; 2002.
3. Mackie DM, Smith ER. From prejudice to intergroup emotions: differentiated reactions to social groups. New York: Psychology Press; 2004.
4. Ponterotto JG, Utsey SO, Pedersen PB. Preventing prejudice: a guide for counselors, educators, and parents, vol. 2. Thousand Oaks: Sage; 2006. p. 3–25.
5. Baker SP, O'Neill B, Haddon Jr W, Long WB. The injury severity score: a method for describing patients with multiple injuries and evaluating emergency care. J Trauma Acute Care Surg. 1974;14(3):187–96.
6. Haider AH, Chang DC, Efron DT, Haut ER, Crandall M, Cornwell EE. Race and insurance status as risk factors for trauma mortality. Arch Surg. 2008;143(10):945–9.
7. Surviving Sepsis Campaign. www.survivingsepsis.org. Accessed 1 Dec 2015.
8. Sepsis. Centers for Disease Control and Prevention. www.cdc.gov/sepsis. Accessed 1 Dec 2015.
9. Esper AM, Moss M, Lewis CA, Nisbet R, Mannino DM, Martin GS. The role of infection and comorbidity: factors that influence disparities in sepsis. Crit Care Med. 2006;34(10):2576–82.
10. Dombrovskiy VY, Martin AA, Sunderram J, Paz HL. Occurrence and outcomes of sepsis: influence of race*. Crit Care Med. 2007;35(3):763–8.
11. Smedley A, Smedley BD. Race as biology is fiction, racism as a social problem is real: anthropological and historical perspectives on the social construction of race. Am Psychol. 2005;60(1):16–26.
12. Jacobellis v. Ohio. 378 US 184.
13. Rachel Dolezal On Being Black: "I didn't deceive anybody" http://www.cnn.com/2015/07/20/us/rachel-dolezal-vanity-fair-feat/. Accessed 1 Dec 2015.
14. Degenholtz HB, Thomas SB, Miller MJ. Race and the intensive care unit: disparities and preferences for end-of-life care. Crit Care Med. 2003;31(5):S373–8.
15. Hauser JM, Kleefield SF, Brennan TA, et al. Minority populations and advance directives: insights from a focus group methodology. Camb Q Healthc Ethics. 1997;6:58–71.

Chapter 10
The Aging Intensivist and Younger Colleagues

Ross Hofmeyr

Introduction

Critical care is an essential but still relatively new discipline with significant clinical, technological, academic and emotional challenges. Younger colleagues entering at training grades have generational differences from the current leadership and require guidance if they are to continue to grow and develop the speciality. Recognising the needs and strengths of younger individuals from various levels of training and age groups allows for better interaction. The interaction with ageing senior intensivists will determine their attitudes towards critical care and their patients. The phases of growth of an intensivist range from initial fear and uncertainty in the novice, through motivation to learn and consolidate knowledge, to challenging older colleagues and finally to consultation and collaboration. The ability of the newer generations to assimilate and remain in touch with the rapid developments in intensive care through the use of technology and social media is a strength which can benefit the entire team. Older colleagues are ideally suited to providing mentorship through teaching, motivation and fostering an environment of collegial scholarship. They benefit in turn from shifting clinical workload, increasing teaching and research outputs and decreasing burnout.

R. Hofmeyr, MBChB, MMed(Anaes), FCA(SA)
Department of Anaesthesia and Perioperative Medicine, Faculty of Health Sciences,
University of Cape Town, Cape Town, South Africa
e-mail: wildmedic@gmail.com

D. Crippen (ed.), *The Intensivist's Challenge: Aging and Career Growth
in a High-Stress Medical Specialty*, DOI 10.1007/978-3-319-30454-0_10

The Interaction of Younger Colleagues with the Ageing Intensivist

Critical care medicine is an undoubtedly essential and entrenched discipline in medicine, but is historically a relatively new speciality [1, 2]. Development of the speciality as a living entity has occurred around the world by parallel evolution. Different models of funding, medical education and oversight have created structurally different critical care services performing the same fundamental purpose: intensive, life-saving medicine for patients requiring organ system support in order to recover from serious illness or injury [3].

Our understanding of disease and the physiological response to insult continues to develop, leading to continuously evolving methods of treatment. As the management of patients changes, so do the demands for the practice of critical care medicine. Accepted wisdom of yesteryear is scorned as pitifully mistaken, and ideas of the future are placed under increasing burdens of evidence as we try to wed the art of care to the science of medicine. Into this shifting milieu, we introduce a workforce which is also changing dynamically over time, generations of practitioners who have differing frames of reference, expectations and learning styles and whose grasp and integration of technology are fundamentally embedded. As one of the author's mentors remarked with regard to patients in ICU, 'If we are not making daily progress, we are falling behind', so too we in the practice of critical care cannot attempt to stem the tide of change but must harness its flow to achieve our immediate goals and those hidden behind the bends of the future.

Phases, Growth and Development in Critical Care

The future intensivist typically first encounters his older colleagues as a trainee or junior doctor. Critical care medicine is a complex interplay of cognitive and clinical skills, and so the development of competence follows the natural progression as described by Burch, from unconscious incompetence to the unconscious competence manifest by senior intensivists, who intuitively recognise the problems and fluidly formulate solutions for complex patients (Table 10.1). The stages of skill development from novice to expert require modifying the input and supervision as the younger colleague gains competence. The entire perception of the disciple will be altered by the manner in which he or she is able to interact with older intensivists. As senior specialists, academics and department heads are likely to be late in their career; their influence on their juniors can have a profound influence on the future of the speciality [4].

Initial exposure to the modern intensive care unit is undoubtedly daunting, and the first emotions experienced by the neophyte include excitement and fear. Fear can be of causing harm by commission or omission and of being shown to lack of knowledge and skill by seniors and peers. While unmitigated fear is distressing and

Table 10.1 Progression of skills in critical care

	Stage of competence	Stage of development	Description
Junior	Unconscious incompetence	Novice	Minimal experience in the critical care environment Task and rule oriented Protocol driven Close supervision required Practical teaching essential *Knowledge acquisition*
	Conscious incompetence	Junior	Recognises limited knowledge and skills and actively engages in learning Applies critical thinking skills Able to formulate a plan Makes use of senior guidance *Knowledge consolidation*
	Conscious competence	Proficient	Able to see entire clinical picture Experience to recognise deviation from expected clinical course *Knowledge refinement*
	Unconscious competence	Expert	Intuitively recognises problems can fluidly integrate and synthesise complex solutions Able to teach critical thinking *Knowledge creation*
Senior			

Adapted from Burch, Hom [5] and Buffum and Brandon [6]

destructive, a small measure may indeed provide the initial motivation for rapid learning. Indeed, this is a fundamental feature of the Socratic method of teaching in medicine, which remains well preserved during teaching rounds in critical care. Therefore, the wise older intensivist will place juniors under a small measure of stress – *eu*stress, improving productivity, rather than *dis*tress – in order to stimulate the learning environment.

Under appropriate guidance, fear is rapidly replaced by respect and motivation to learn. The junior colleague recognises the knowledge and clinical skill of his senior and seeks to emulate this behaviour and competence. At this point, the emphasis of the older intensivist must be to act as an ideal role model; emphasis on ideal care and structured decision-making is essential. Integration of theoretical learning into clinical practice and consolidation of clinical skills are essential.

The next phase for the developing intensivist is heralded by the novice beginning to challenge the older intensivist. While this may seem presumptuous or adversarial at first, it should be recognised as a positive step. In order to challenge the senior's opinions, the young intensivist must have been studying, reading the literature or seeking other sources of education in critical care. These are ideal moments for teaching, for either the ageing intensivist can defend his position eloquently or must reconsider the veracity of his knowledge. This is the time to actively encourage the younger colleague to research and present his/her arguments, as the entire team is likely to benefit.

An important watershed in the career of the young intensivists occurs when they become independent specialists. While able to practise without senior oversight, an organisational culture should be created in which they feel free to openly consult about challenging cases or difficult decisions. This allows ongoing learning and protects the young specialist against inadvertent errors.

The final stages of a career in critical care commence when the younger colleague begins to be challenged by juniors himself. The emphasis shifts gradually from being a protégé to becoming a mentor. The now established intensivist should recognise that this is a natural progression, and while it is natural to feel threatened by these challenges, it is a crucial aspect of the development of both the speciality and the next generation of critical care physicians. Finally, it behoves the individual to recognise that they themselves are becoming ageing intensivists and gradually alter their practice to allow for their changing capabilities.

Generational Differences and Embracing Technology

The changes in the attitudes, expectations and behaviour of staff as generations pass must be understood and integrated into this model. Strategies for training and practice in intensive care that functioned well for the past generations can and will not work in the future. Many of the technologies that our next generation of juniors will use – and the clinical work that they will undertake – do not yet exist or have not yet been integrated into medicine.

The current leadership in critical care on an international and individual unit basis consists heavily of members of the "Mature" and "Boomer" generations. A strong ethos of personal responsibility, while putting the needs of the patient and institution first, permeates these generations, with respect for hierarchy and the creation of robust structures heavily valued. However, these generations are nearing and reaching retirement and are steadily being replaced by Generations X and Y (the latter also known "Generation Next" or "Millennials"), born between 1980 and 2000 [6].

Now in their 30s, Gen X doctors are the new intensivists, raised with high expectations of themselves and others, technologically savvy and independently driven but expecting ongoing two-way communication. At least in the First World, the Millennials are effortlessly integrated with technology – at times to the point of reliance – and highly and effective multitaskers but have been accused of requiring continuous feedback and affirmation. The wise ageing intensivist will resist neither the desires for dialogue and 360° communication nor the increasing technological integration of the younger generations but will rather culture and encourage these teaching opportunities. The changing lifestyle demands of younger colleagues will require revision of management strategies and a shift in the staffing paradigms but will ensure the longevity of the speciality and dedication of younger generations.

Two prime examples of the value of technology and communication integration for collegial interaction are the Critical Care Mailing List (CCM-L) curated by the editor of this volume, and the incredible growth and expansion of the #FOAMed movement. CCM-L [7] is well described elsewhere, having developed in the era in which e-mail was the most rapid and effective method of idea dissipation and sharing between colleagues [8]. Today, while traditional mailing lists are still in use, the epitome of integrated online knowledge sharing is the #FOAMed community. An acronym for 'free open-access medical education', FOAMed comprises an interlinked community of practitioners (heavily represented by emergency medicine and critical care doctors) who use rapid-sharing methods such as Twitter and medical blogs to discuss the latest developments and disseminate ideas [9]. While strongly criticised for a lack of formal peer review, the immediacy of the discourse and accessibility of colleagues around the world has greatly strengthened the learning and practice of practitioners who have embraced the concept [10]. Due to their open attitudes to social media and crowdsourcing of ideas, younger clinicians are more inclined to make use of these resources. The savvy older intensivist will encourage the academic nature of these pursuits while positively guiding their juniors to understand what comprises appropriate and inappropriate use.

Mentorship

In the *Odyssey*, Homer describes how Odysseus assigns his old friend Mentor to take charge of the education of Odysseus's son Telemachus, while he campaigns in the Trojan War. In his absence, the goddess Athena takes the form of Mentor to enhance his spiritual and emotional development. The term *mentor* has thus come to denote a senior colleague who forms a personal professional relationship (and often lasting friendship) with his or her *protégé* in order to impart wisdom, knowledge, skill and attitudes. Rather than a simple advisory role, this relationship also recognises and addresses the emotional well-being of the protégé. The field of critical care medicine, where academically challenging concepts are infused with the dilemmas and emotions of life-changing and life-ending decisions, is ideally suited to mentorship by experienced intensivists.

The author attributes his interest in (and passion for) acute-phase critical care to a series of astute mentors. As a medical student with a great interest in trauma care, it would have been easy to be sidelined as an 'adrenaline junkie', but a senior with foresight was able to challenge the energy into modest research and extra clinical experience. This resulted in forays into academic writing and involvement in trauma teaching. Later, in a modest regional hospital setting with severe resource limitations, a set of mentors cultivated a strong ethos of unashamedly campaigning for improved standards of care. In addition to significant personal growth, this resulted in tangible benefits to patients and early-career publication.

Seven roles have been proposed for the mentor-physician: teacher, sponsor, advisor, agent, role model, coach and confidant [11]. Each of these is applicable in the field of critical care medicine, and the ageing intensivist is ideally suited to providing this role. Indeed, formal mentoring programmes in critical care have been established in several centres and under the auspices of the professional societies.

The role of teacher is obvious but should not focus purely on the transmission of facts, for these may be obtained in any relevant reference. Rather, teaching must centre upon the acquisition of critical learning skills and an attitude towards ongoing learning. The skilled mentor imparts the facets of critical thinking by stimulating analysis and discussion.

Sponsorship is critical. The protégé must be introduced to other colleagues who will ultimately form a support network (either for academic advancement or clinical purposes) through open discussion and constructive criticism. An astute mentor will recognise the partnerships which play to the strengths of the protégé: research, teaching, collaboration on clinical guidelines, etc.

As an advisor, the mentor in critical care serves as more than an academic guide. This role encompasses providing counsel that the young intensivist lacks through inexperience. The mentor can share historical narrative which allows the junior to create his own solutions, rather than simply providing an answer. The protégé models his *behaviour* on the mentor, instead of blindly applying rote solutions. In response to recognising appropriate engagement, the mentor acts as an agent, introducing the protégé to suitable opportunities for career growth.

Perhaps the most critical purpose of a mentor is that of a role model. Responsibility and work ethic in critical care are seldom effectively taught but are perfectly demonstrated by the older generation of intensivists. The junior doctor will be strongly influenced by the work ethic of the mentor, by his or her manner with patients and other colleagues and by patterns of clinical decision-making. While mentorship does not require infallibility, it does carry a burden or responsibility for setting a worthy example. The hypocrisy of mentor who does not practise what he preaches will be rapidly recognised and undermine the relationship. A junior colleague will take careful note of his senior's moral decisions, as these cannot be taught outside of a clinical environment.

A coach's responsibility is to train his players, but he will be measured on their success. In the presence of requisite skill, success is determined by motivation. As a coach, the mentor feeds this motivation through inspiration. For clinical work in intensive care, this involves demonstrating that surmounting the challenges of diagnosis and management brings a sense of satisfaction and success. In research, the inspiration is curiosity; the mentor must encourage the junior colleague to keep questioning until the limit of knowledge is reached and then to devise ways of pushing beyond this point through new studies. A good coach will recognise and praise performance and then set a further and higher goal.

As Cherry-Garrard wrote, 'The mutual conquest of difficulties is the cement of friendship' [12]. Certainly, critical care provides ample difficulties. As a confidante, the ageing intensivist can share and explore the emotional responses – fear, frustration, heartache, loss, success, joy – and ensure that the younger colleague understands that these feelings are natural. Older colleagues help the young intensivist to recognise and validate their emotions by not appearing emotionless and unaffected but rather admitting to emotion. Reflecting on difficult decisions, expressing empathy and showing behaviours which illustrate that they are also affected by the challenges of critical care help younger colleagues to become balanced specialists. By providing a supportive and confidential ear, an experienced colleague also gains the trust required to be heard attentively when the protégé requires rebuke and guidance. Through the mentorship role, the ageing intensivist can demonstrate how to achieve a balance between professional pursuits and home life that prevents burnout.

It is vital to understand that mentorship is not a unidirectional process. The protégé most certainly benefits immensely from guidance and input, but the mentor benefits through more than reflected success. Shifting the burden of clinical workload, increasing research and publication output, delegating administrative tasks and gradually generating capacity to hand over leadership roles all benefit the mentor. The senior is able to learn by proxy, as the energy and technological integration of the younger colleague will undoubtedly unearth new material. Ultimately, the growth of the discipline will be ensured through effective mentorship.

Shifting Focus and Roles for Ageing Intensivists

The literature on workplace performance during ageing is clear. Fluid thinking, memory, processing speed, visual and hearing acuity and manual dexterity decrease with age, while verbal skills and semantic capability is often well preserved. Ageing doctors are often skilled in both diagnosis through experience and pattern recognition, and their aptitude for oration and teaching are excellent [13]. Declining stamina for after-hours work is well balanced by an aptitude for supervision and wealth of experience that is ideally suited for supervising research, mentoring, teaching activities, etc. The wise young intensivist will retain positions and roles in his or her unit for the involvement of the ageing colleague, whose experience and perspective will enrich the environment for all concerned.

> Watch out for those coming up behind you. You may well be one of their mentors;
> they just haven't told you yet.
> Rebecca Smith,
> 'Making the Most of your Mentor'[14]

References

1. Vincent JL. Critical care–where have we been and where are we going? Crit Care. 2013;17 Suppl 1:S2.
2. Bryan-Brown CW. My first 50 years of critical care (1956–2006). Am J Crit Care. 2007;16(1):12–6.
3. Crippen DE. ICU resource allocation in the new millennium. 1st ed. New York: Springer; 2013. 351 p.
4. Wood LD. Mentorship in pulmonary and critical care medicine. Am J Respir Crit Care Med. 2010;182(10):1215–6.

5. Hom EM. Coaching and mentoring new graduates entering perinatal nursing practice. J Perinat Neonatal Nurs. 2003;17(1):35–49.
6. Buffum AR, Brandon DH. Mentoring new nurses in the neonatal intensive care unit: impact on satisfaction and retention. J Perinat Neonatal Nurs. 2009;23(4):357–62.
7. Crippen D. CCM-L [Mailing List]. [cited 2015 30 November 2015]. Available from: https://list.pitt.edu/mailman/listinfo/ccm-l.
8. Crippen D. CCM-L: the International Internet Critical Care Medicine Group: BookCrafters. 144 p.
9. Nickson C. FOAM 2014 [cited 2015 30 November 2015]. Available from: http://lifeinthe fastlane.com/foam/.
10. Thoma B, Chan T, Desouza N, Lin M. Implementing peer review at an emergency medicine blog: bridging the gap between educators and clinical experts. CJEM. 2015;17(2):188–91.
11. Tobin MJ. Mentoring: seven roles and some specifics. Am J Respir Crit Care Med. 2004;170(2):114–7.
12. Cherry-Garrard A. The Worst Journey in the World 1922.
13. Skowronski GA, Peisah C. The greying intensivist: ageing and medical practice – everyone's problem. Med J Aust. 2012;196(8):505–7.
14. Smith R. Making the Most of Your Mentor www.cicm.org.au: College of Intensive Care Medicine of Australia and New Zealand; [cited 2015 30 November 2015]. Available from: http://www.cicm.org.au/Newsletters/Trainee-Newsletter/Archive/July-2015/Making-the-Most-of-your-Mentor.

Chapter 11
Nearing the Clinical End:
A Female Perspective

Marie R. Baldisseri

> *"Medicine is so broad a field, so closely interwoven with general interests…that it must be regarded as one of those great departments of work in which the cooperation of men and women is needed to fulfill all its requirements".*
>
> *Dr. Elizabeth Blackwell, a leading public health activist who graduated first in her class and became the first woman in the world to receive a medical degree in 1849 in the USA*

How I Got Here

"Where to start?" is a ubiquitous and rather annoying question when asked to give opinions about oneself. "Should I tell you my life story?" "Do you want to hear how I could have done it differently?" "Shall I tell you my regrets or my successes?" "Does the information I tell you ultimately make a difference in your life choices and your personal odyssey?" The questions could go on, but I'll choose to give you my truths from a retrospect of 28 years of professional life, 30 years of married life, and 60 years of "being female." In my opinion, none of these questions is more important or dominates the other – my professional life, my married life, my years as a mother of three children, and my life as a woman make up who am I. I could not imagine *becoming me* or *being me* – having one without the other.

I came from a solid and loving family with a dad who was a professional. Both my parents came from very modest backgrounds. They were the son and daughter of Irish and Italian immigrants. My parents disagreed on many issues over the years, but the sole idea that cemented their relationship was their unflagging belief that education was the key to advancement in life. Their immigrant parents had believed that hard work was the answer to the American dream, which was to make money so you could provide for your children and have a better life than they did. My parents took it a step further. They believed that hard work alone in America might

M.R. Baldisseri, MD, MPH, FCCM
Department of Critical Care Medicine, University of Pittsburgh Medical Center,
Pittsburgh, PA, USA
e-mail: Baldisserimr@ccm.upmc.edu

© Springer International Publishing Switzerland 2016
D. Crippen (ed.), *The Intensivist's Challenge: Aging and Career Growth in a High-Stress Medical Specialty*, DOI 10.1007/978-3-319-30454-0_11

not get you that pot of gold at the end of the rainbow. Despite not having the necessary means and having to take out several loans to pay tuition at private elementary and high schools, colleges, and finally medical school and graduate school for my sister and I, nothing was too high a price for them to make sure we got the most out of the educational system that would allow us to live out the American dream.

I knew my parents ideas about schooling and I since I was one of the smart kids at school, their plan gelled with mine pretty well. However, I was somewhat clueless as to what my parents had truly envisioned for me. I liked people, found it easy to talk to them, and had a compassionate streak, so I thought nursing would be a noble pursuit. I remember when I was about 13 years old and my mom asked me what I wanted to be when I grew up. My secret wish was to be a journalist or an FBI detective, but I had already figured out that they weren't going to be too pleased with either of those choices. Instead, I told my mom that I wanted to be a nurse. I thought this would be the perfect profession for someone who was smart, compassionate, and hardworking (even then I had an inflated view of myself). She looked at me for probably a few seconds and said, "Why do you want to be a nurse?" "Do you want to take orders or give them?" I figured she recognized that I could be pushy and bossy, and she was implying that being a nurse wouldn't totally appease those traits. I don't think she was being pejorative or denigrating toward nurses. In fact, it had been her own personal dream to be a nurse when she was younger. However, she knew my personality, and even more importantly, she expected me to choose a career with a graduate degree because that's the highest you can achieve in school. It was that simple for her. She told me in no uncertain terms, "If you love medicine so much, be a doctor – this way you get to give the orders, rather than follow them." She followed up by saying, "If you don't want medicine, then be a lawyer or engineer." In her mind, they were the best and only choices I could and should make. It sounded rather reasonable to a 13-year-old with an overinflated ego, so I took her advice and decided to be a physician.

My trek began painfully so at first. I simply wasn't as smart as most of the people who wanted to be docs in the USA (a very bitter pill to swallow at the time) or at least that's what I believed of myself for many years. I didn't get accepted to an American medical school on my first attempt, even after receiving my first master's degree in biomedical sciences, which I was sure would give me a heads up on other candidates. While my parents pushed me to not abandon my "dream" (or was it theirs?), they encouraged me to look outside the USA to attend medical school. I finished at a phenomenal foreign medical school in Spain and was then accepted after completing medical school to a reasonably good internal medicine training program in one of the most underserved – not to mention one of the most dangerous – neighborhoods in Brooklyn, Bedford Stuyvesant. It was then I really went into overdrive. I know it sounds rather trite, but I was set on being the very best and accomplish what it took to be at the top. I literally worked my butt off, got accepted at the best critical care training program in the world at the University of Pittsburgh, and thought I had it made it to the big time. Well, not quite yet.

Specialty training in critical care medicine after residency was simply tortuous. It had nothing to do with my educational background or my gender – that never was an issue during residency or fellowship where men and women were treated rather equally. The workload and the call schedule during my critical care fellowship were beyond imagination. My night calls were every two to three nights, and most of what I remember from my fellowship is just being tired continuously although the reality was that I was uber-trained in critical care medicine! I had just gotten married a few months before I came to Pittsburgh and rarely saw my husband during my first year of fellowship. He was completing additional fellowship training in cardiology, and the reality was that we were both incredibly busy. It wasn't how I imagined my first year of marriage would be – long walks in the park, candlelight dinners, and endless nights of unbridled passion…you get the picture. The reality was rather different. I chose to sleep every opportunity that I got. Despite our frenetic schedules, though, we were very happy. However, we never considered starting a family under such circumstances.

So why did I choose critical care medicine as my future endeavor? It's a loaded question. I finished my residency in 1985, and at that time, critical care was a barely recognized field of medicine. My husband, who was a fellow in cardiology around the same time I was completing my residency, and many of my professional colleagues and friends told me in no uncertain terms that there was simply no future for me in critical care. They advised me to change my career path if I planned to have a productive career in medicine both educationally and financially. (Side note – "Do any female physicians actually meet anyone but other physicians?" In my generation, the answer was "Not really." I certainly didn't have much of a social life back then, and the reality was that my colleagues and friends in the hospital were my only social contacts. It's probably pertinent at this point to mention that the HIV/AIDS epidemic was just beginning to be recognized, and "good girls" like me weren't frequenting the NYC bars, where, according to the media, we were likely to catch the fatal disease.) Critical care medicine was a novel idea, but the surgeons and pulmonary docs weren't going to give up their ICUs to a group of so-called ICU docs. Even back in the 1980s, we were the new kids on the block, and the practice of critical care was still unheard of in many places. Naturally, I chose to ignore my loved one's well-intentioned advice, primarily because there was absolutely no other field that excited me both intellectually and procedurally as ICU medicine. I had found the perfect profession – and it was literally an epiphany for me. On the first day of my ICU rotation as an intern, the ICU was frenetic with multiple admissions, patients coding, and general mayhem. I decided on that very day that the chaos, the intellectual stimulation, and the role of being a "detective" in trying to assess critically ill patients and figure out their diagnosis (my chance to be Jodi Foster, as an FBI detective, in the movie, "Silence of the Lambs") were perfect for me. I found where I needed to be – what I was really good at – and I haven't looked back since.

Over the years, the question of why I chose critical care medicine from the perspective of being a *female* physician has come up innumerable times by female college students, medical students, and residents. *Why choose a field where it's assumed that the days will be long and night and weekend calls in the hospital will be inevitable?* For many young women, this remains a germane issue and can be a deal breaker. *Why choose a field of medicine that limits time for leisure or time to raise a family?* That question has really never changed over the years, but I have distinctly noticed a change in women's expectations for themselves over time – women have gradually taken more and more on themselves. They expect to have full-time jobs, get married, have a family, and are the "perfect" wife, mom, and professional. Obviously, there are many socioeconomic and geopolitical reasons why women have adapted this view. The liberated woman decided she could do it all. Gradually, society began to expect this practice as the norm. It's a wonderful concept in my eyes, but the reality is that the field of critical care medicine is a tough one, emotionally and physically. As a female, it's simply harder. It has little to do with the job, in my opinion, but directly relates to the fact that as caregivers for our kids, oftentimes the bulk of the chores and tasks of raising children falls to the woman. There are exceptions, of course, but how can you not sign your child up for the music lessons, the sport games, and the dance classes? In almost every relationship I know where both parents are physicians or other professionals, the mom is usually the one who spends more time bringing the kids to sporting events, birthday parties, school functions, etc. Going to work each day to a hectic, fast-paced, emotionally wrenching job was a calming experience compared to raising a family. I have a wonderful husband who helped as much as he could; nonetheless, the stress of those early years (along with the utter joys of motherhood, of course) still makes me wonder, "How did I manage to do it all?" I'm not sure how I made it through those years unscarred. A combination of a loving husband, a wonderful secretary, friends, and nurses who helped me as often as they could, and parents who, although they lived a good distance away in Rhode Island, would drop everything to come to Pittsburgh to give us a break and allow us some precious time together without the kids made our lives manageable. But the day-to-day existence was not easy on many fronts.

I'm at the Top

Ok not surprisingly, I made it through my 2-year fellowship in critical care, and I was then offered an attending position at the University. *Now,* I finally felt like I got my foot in the door of academia. What I wasn't quite as prepared for was the lack of women in my department. For almost 10 years, I was the only woman or one of two in a very large department of male ICU physicians. I was a surgical ICU physician, and most of the surgeons were male. I found after some time that working with men was not very different than working with women. It wasn't always pleasant, and there were moments of tears, frustration, and anger, particularly when dealing with surgeons on a day-to-day basis. One of my favorite anecdotes is about a fellow intensivist in my department when I was a junior attending. My chairman had just announced at a faculty meeting that I was pregnant and would have to take a few weeks off from clinical service, so the rest of the department members would have to cover my ICU time. There was a moment of stunned silence, and the first question asked by one of my colleagues was "She is going to pay us back for the time we cover for her, right?" "How long do we have to do this for?" At the time, I was furious with these comments, but over the years, I even learned to laugh off this incident. I now realize that these comments weren't malicious and that my colleagues weren't evil misogynists. Most of them simply had not worked with women in the past, and this was uncharted territory for them.

I learned very quickly that although some might not like your gender, you must use your knowledge to influence and convince practitioners in medicine and surgery. Even the most prejudicial and biased physician or surgeon will usually acquiesce when your argument beats his based on evidence in the literature. Although I've always been uncomfortable with confrontations, I gradually learned to stand my ground when I had to and push back when I believed it was the best thing to do for the patient. I never saw my interactions as a battle of the sexes but rather as a "robust" exchange of ideas. Interestingly though, some of the most contentious practitioners, luckily there were very few of them, that I met over the years have been women, not men. It's been my impression that these women felt they had to prove themselves to others and being overbearing (or sometimes downright rude) was their way to cope with the stress of their professional and personal lives. I've always felt disappointed interacting with these women. Over the years, I've learned that a smile, a laugh, or solid data usually convinces people more easily. Unfortunately, rude and contentious men don't experience this same type of prejudice. Instead, they are usually described as just being "demanding" – as if that is a trait that one should be envious of.

On my journey, I had to make some painful career decisions. I was ambitious and planned to rise in my department. I had already been promoted to medical director of two ICUs and envisioned a greater administrative role for myself in the department. However, my kids had grown into preteens and teenagers. I saw how other parents struggled with their teenagers – some had lost the battle to drugs, alcohol, and just plain indifference. I was determined that was not going to happen to our kids. This meant that I had to make a choice – it was my decision to cut down on my clinical time in the ICU and work part-time. I remember when I told the chairman of the department that was my plan. He looked at me and said it had never been done before. I couldn't believe my response: "It's either a part-time position or I will have to quit and leave for good." I had done everything to get to this pinnacle in my career and was now actually considering letting it all slip away. I held my breath when he reconsidered and then exhaled when he smiled and said "Why not? There's always a first time for everything." Whether he made that decision because he thought I was too valuable to the department or whether he just didn't want to go through the hassle of having to redo the clinical schedule with one less faculty member, I didn't know and frankly didn't care. But I like to think it was the former.

For the next 28 years of my career, I was a teacher and a clinician not only as a university faculty member but internationally as well. As a popular speaker on critical care topics, I found myself repeatedly invited to many countries worldwide.

My extensive travels *influenced my growing interests in global health and disaster medicine. I wanted to* make a difference in improving the delivery of critical care in resource-limited venues. I learned that critically ill patients can be adequately managed without sophisticated technology, and simple basic protocols, guidelines, and checklists are valuable tools in many of the poorer countries. Trained as a physician, my focus has always been on the individual patient; my journey into public/global health taught me that improvement must come at the level of populations. To broaden my knowledge base in global health, I decided to go back to school and obtain my MPH at Johns Hopkins – that was a challenge since I was still working at the same time. I was able to start my own nonprofit organization dedicated to educational and clinical care in the fields of critical care and disaster medicine worldwide. I would never have imagined that in addition to my clinical life, I would have another professional life which has given me a chance to see the world as a global citizen.

Although I had chosen not to become deeply involved with an administrative role in my own department, I became increasingly involved with my professional medical society. It's been a wonderful experience being associated with a professional society with so many eclectic members but who all share a love of critical care. The number of women in our society has continued to increase over time, and as a member, I have advanced far beyond what I had hoped for, as a national and international speaker and ultimately as the chancellor of the American College of Critical Care Medicine. Among my professional colleagues in the society, I really don't believe that I've ever experienced the bias and prejudice which I know are clearly more prevalent in other professional medical societies.

I now truly feel comfortable in my expertise and my skills in those roles after 28 years of countless local, regional, national, and international lectures, ICU rounding, and bedside teaching of students, residents, and fellows. I have reached the stage in my career where I am confident in my skills and knowledge as a critical care clinician and teacher. I chose my career well. Being unsure whether I was going to excel in a profession where there are so many intellectual giants, many of whom work in my department, I know now that I'm at the top of my game, and it just feels great.

Am I Going to Hit Bottom?

What is the most recent data of women in medicine, for those in critical care medicine, and of those who are approaching that "golden age" they refer to so euphemistically? For the year 2013–2014, the number of females in medicine and surgery continued to increase comprising 36 % of the physician workforce in the USA with 47 % as medical students and 46 % as residents [1]. The percentage of women in the specialty of pulmonary and critical care medicine comprises 26.8 % and those over the age of 55 years of age approximates 36 % [1]. Among Asians, blacks or African-Americans, and Hispanics or Latinos, women make up a greater percentage of younger physicians (age 29 and younger). Among white physicians in 2013, a greater percentage of those from all age ranges were men, compared to women. The greatest disparity between white men and women exists among physicians age 50–64 [2]. The AAMC reported in 2010 that as a specialty, critical care medicine had one of the lowest percentages of women at 16.8 % with almost 40 % of them age 55 or older [3]. Specialties with lower percentages than critical care included all the different surgical specialties and cardiology.

Now that I'm at the pinnacle of my career, there are only two options for me from here on out – I could plateau for a time or I start the downward spiral into oblivion. I'm hoping this phase of greatness lasts a while, but there's this little voice in my head saying, "You can't be here forever." "Why can't you remember the little things anymore?" "Why are you so mentally and physically exhausted when you come home from work each day that you reach for that one glass of red wine and zone out in front of the TV"? The upside is that I wake up every day eager and anxious to go to work to see what new patients were admitted overnight wondering what new challenges and diagnostic mysteries the day will bring. At times, I think I've seen it all, and then a new patient comes in and I'm completely baffled as to what's wrong with them. It takes time, energy, and effort to make the right diagnosis, and I feel young all over again.

I've had a blessed and fortuitous life. For many years as an international lecturer, I've traveled to innumerable foreign cities, observing the different practices of critical care. I've become particularly interested in critical care globally and disaster medicine. Many years ago, I decided to start my own foundation and have been able to teach about critical care and disaster medicine all over the world. Fortuitously, this may be my answer to "retirement." I can't imagine retiring at the (young) age of 60, but I know realistically, it's not too far off. My professional life has defined who I am for so long; it's frightening to think of what else is out there I could do. I've been associated with a top-rated university program for decades. What happens when it's just me and I'm not representing my department anymore? I don't believe that my life as a teacher will stop anytime soon – whether it's as a department member, an invited speaker, or working for my foundation. My life as a clinician is less predetermined in terms of the number of years when I can work as hard as I do now. There's a reason why you don't see many older intensivists. The simple truth is that it is a demanding job. Younger physicians, although not as experienced or as adept in the ICU, simply have a higher level of energy that gets them through the strenuous days and nights.

As a woman and mother of three young adults, I have to consider that in the next few years (TBD), I may become a grandmother. I can't think of a job I want more. There are a lot of unknowns in my life right now. While there's no pressure to make any immediate changes, I know that within the next 5–10 years, I have to make some very hard decisions. Many of my friends and colleagues have hit that magical age of retirement and are happy. My greatest fear is that I will have to give up something I love, but as a mother, a wife, and a woman, there are so many lovely options out there for me. Fear of what's to come is silly – a different chapter awaits me.

"I do think that when it comes to aging, we're held to a different standard than men. Some guy said to me: "Don't you think you're too old to sing rock n' roll?" I said: "You'd better check with Mick Jagger".

Cher, Fifty on Fifty: Wisdom, Inspiration, and Reflections on Women's Lives Well Lived by Bonnie Miller Rubin, November 1998

References

1. AMN® Healthcare. Women in medicine: a review of changing physician demographics, female physicians by specialty, state and related data. 2015. https://www.amnhealthcare.com/upload-edFiles/MainSite/Content/Staffing_Recruitment/Staffcare-WP-Women%20in%20Med.pdf.
2. AAMC 2013 State Physician Workforce Data Book. https://www.aamc.org/download/362168/data/2013statephysicianworkforcedatabook.pdf.
3. AAMC 2012 Physician Specialty Data Book. https://www.aamc.org/download/313228/data/2012physicianspecialtydatabook.pdf.

Chapter 12
Good Times, Bad Times, Time to Get Out Alive: Ruminations of a Retiring Critical Care Physician

Mark A. Mazer

> *"Beneath a lover's moon, I'm waiting*
> *I am the pilot of the storm*
> *Adrift in pleasure I may drown*
> *I built this ship, it is my making*
> *And furthermore my self-control*
> *I can't rely on anymore"*
>
> "Ship of Fools," Robert Plant

Preparation for a career in critical care medicine started from the onset of my internal medicine residency during the early 1980s. Whereas I greatly enjoyed the intellectual challenges presented by patients on the general medical ward, I quickly grew to appreciate the cognitive as well as the direct hands-on skills needed to care for the most critically ill patients. The attending staff rewarded my passion by allowing me to do elective rotations in the intensive care unit, as well as offering instruction in advanced resuscitation techniques.

As a senior medical resident, my interaction with the nursing staff concerning the care of one particular patient was extremely formative. The young man was mechanically ventilated for an atypical pneumonia. There were needle tracks on his extremities, and he was afflicted by a newly described disease characterized by chronic wasting, diarrhea, and lymphadenopathy. Little was known about this condition; therefore, much apprehension was prevalent among healthcare workers concerning this patient. The nursing staff was hesitant to enter the room of this extremely ill gentleman.

I emerged from the call room after having read an article concerning the use of trimethoprim-sulfa for the treatment of atypical pneumonia caused by *Pneumocystis carinii* in intravenous drug users. Colorful images of *Pneumocystis* trophozoites were still fresh in my mind's eye as I donned protective gear outside the patient's

M.A. Mazer, MD
Department of Critical Care Medicine, Vidant Medical Center,
600 Moye Boulevard, Greenville, NC 27834, USA
e-mail: mazerm@ecu.edu; mmazer@suddenlink.net

© Springer International Publishing Switzerland 2016
D. Crippen (ed.), *The Intensivist's Challenge: Aging and Career Growth in a High-Stress Medical Specialty*, DOI 10.1007/978-3-319-30454-0_12

room. An inquisitive group of nurses huddled outside the room, and someone asked what I was doing. I commented on the article and opined that it would be a shame for this young man to die without a trial of trimethoprim-sulfa. I proffered this remark with curiosity to note what effect it would have on the nursing staff. Then I entered the room, made a deliberate gesture to pull back the sheets, and reexamined the patient. Several nurses entered the room soon thereafter to join me. Afterward I was gratified to note a team of nurses huddled inside the patient's room, with the newly prescribed antibiotic coursing into his veins.

This episode had a deep effect on me. I recognized that my words, supplemented by appropriate behavior, could have a profound effect on other healthcare providers. The realization came that I was destined to have a career in intensive care medicine, not only as a clinician but also as an educator and leader.

I felt out of place prior to my interview for a critical care fellowship at the National Institutes of Health. The waiting room was otherwise packed with tense, well-groomed candidates from prestigious training programs. Dressed in khaki pants, a worn shirt, an unremarkable tie, and no dress coat, I stuck out like a sore thumb. However, the Deputy Chief of Critical Care Medicine, Dr. Henry Masur, sporting casual pants and a loose tie, immediately put me at ease. I accompanied him to the microbiology laboratory to review stains of bronchoalveolar lavage fluid obtained from a patient with community-acquired cellular immune deficiency and pneumonia. He placed a specimen slide on the stage of a double-headed microscope and invited me to comment. Peering through the lenses, I rejoined without hesitation that *Pneumocystis carinii* trophozoites were clearly visible and that the patient might benefit from trimethoprim-sulfa. Dr. Masur peered at me over the microscope and asked why I was so confident. After recounting my recent experience with a similar patient, he jested that if I could find my way back to his office alone while he tended to a few other matters, I would have a spot in the program.

During the early to mid-1980s, the first wave of formally trained critical care physicians graduated and set out to practice. Though the pioneers of critical care medicine realized the benefits of staffing intensive care units with dedicated practitioners, the general medical community was yet to be convinced. During my interview for a position with an academic community hospital in Georgia, the chief of staff quipped he was not convinced of the need to hire someone with my training, though it might nevertheless be beneficial. Later an employee of the Georgia State Board of Medicine called to inquire what a critical care physician does. She subsequently informed to me that I was the first person with such credentials to apply for licensure in the state. I felt like a pioneer getting ready to explore a brave New World.

During the first decade of my career, I was confronted with incredulity and passive, if not overt, hostility. The first patient I saw as an attending physician was an elderly lady with dementia. She had suffered a cardiac arrest in a nursing facility and remained comatose 1 week after the event. Her family practitioner, a kind-appearing, gray-haired, bespectacled gentleman asked if I would not mind assessing his patient. She was otherwise being managed by a pulmonologist, cardiologist, nephrologist, infectious disease specialist, neurologist, and an endocrinologist.

After examining the patient, I emerged from the room and informed my new colleague that his patient was deceased. The friendly smile dissipated and he asked me to clarify. I detailed her neurologic examination which was compatible with death by neurological criteria.

"What next?" he queried, with a confused look on his face.

"The State of Georgia recognizes death by neurologic criteria. The next step is a formal apnea test. If she does not breath, we should declare her formally deceased," I answered.

"What about the heartbeat on the monitor?" he asked apprehensively.

"The heart will stop beating after ventilator support is withdrawn," I replied.

He closed her chart, stood up from his chair, and looked at me with resignation and sighed.

"Do what needs to be done young man. What you're getting ready to do is against my religion, but thank you very much."

Ironically, after all the years of rigorous training, my first formal patient encounter as an attending physician was not to resuscitate, rather to deescalate and withdraw aggressive measures from a deceased person on a mechanical ventilator. In many ways, this very first encounter was a paradigm of my subsequent career.

I was treated to a somewhat frosty reaction from some of the other consultants. Young and naïve, I was taken aback by some of their vituperative comments. It was a rude awakening to realize that medicine is not always practiced for the benefit of the patient, but sometimes only for shameless financial gain. Only one day on the job and struggles with ethical issues and conflict with colleagues were just beginning. The first decade of my critical care career was characterized by dogged and often belittled efforts to establish myself as a credible medical practitioner. Critical care medicine had not yet been recognized as a valid subspecialty of internal medicine, and this symbolized the resistance and prejudice of the general medical community at large. On the bright side, many colleagues did come to appreciate my efforts; their encouragement and gratification relating to patient care generally outweighed these frustrations.

Our well-intended mentors apparently had no idea of the frigid reception waiting the initial wave of critical care physicians as we struggled to integrate with other acute care practitioners. Who were we to perform procedures such as endotracheal intubation, mechanical ventilator management, central line, arterial line and pulmonary artery catheter insertion, and renal replacement therapy? All too often I was dressed down unabashedly by other consultants in front of patients and families and accused of overstepping my bounds. However, not one patient, family, or nurse ever complained while I was actively intervening during a crisis, and their approving smiles, winks, and nods during such tirades were more than enough to encourage me to pursue my path. Though residual pockets of resistance remain to this day, critical care medicine is finally a bona fide subspecialty, and its practitioners are well respected and integrated into the continuum of care. In retrospect, I am extremely gratified to have been a foot soldier in these early battles to establish critical care medicine on equal footing with other subspecialties. However, reflecting back on my career, these conflicts exacted an enormous personal and emotional toll.

I have immeasurably enjoyed the practice of critical care medicine which has offered me satisfaction and fulfillment on many different levels. I have had the opportunity to save lives, orchestrate peaceful death, and help families go on despite immense tragedy. I continue to have the honor and privilege of teaching medical students, residents, fellows, advanced practitioners, nurses, and other allied health professionals. During the course of my career, I have overcome obstacles and established, structured, and organized successful critical care delivery systems in four different hospitals. These achievements have been uplifting and exhilarating.

However, there is a dark side which has become increasingly overwhelming and oppressive. Thirty years of struggle with a broken healthcare system catering to a death-denying society has taken an irreparable emotional toll. Though incredibly long hours and endless strings of sleepless nights have certainly been taxing, cumulative physical fatigue and sleep deprivation have not worn me down to the point of contemplating retirement.

Of all the challenges and frustrations I regularly confront, none are more onerous than dealing with the consequences of appalling, irresponsible lack of realistic end-of-life planning all too often evident during the penultimate moments of life. The emotional burden of dealing with unprepared patients and families, consequent to this egregious breach of fundamental fiduciary medical responsibility, is the *primum movens* of my decision to eventually eschew clinical practice.

As practitioners gathered cumulative clinical experience, the practical limits of critical care progressively became apparent. Consequent to the evolving awareness of the nebulous notion of futility, and attempts to precisely identify patients not likely to benefit from critical care, emerged an extraordinary sequence of ethical conundrums. These fundamental ethical issues continue to command debate among clinicians, ethicists, religious authority, and the public. Further, the legal system had to evolve in recognition of the practical limits of critical care therapies. My career started not long after the Quinlan case clarified the fundamental difference between killing and allowing a patient to die a natural death in the wake of withholding artificial life support [1]. Thereafter, Nancy Cruzan's legal voyage culminated in the Presidential Right to Self Determination Act and the advent of advance directives [2, 3]. Sadly, far too many medical practitioners, and many in the general public, still continue to harbor unrealistic expectations or purposely ignore the lessons that decades of critical care medicine have taught us.

The field of palliative care medicine has also evolved, due in no small measure to the amassed lessons of critical care. A significant paradigm shift has occurred during my career concerning end-of-life care. In the early years of my career, most patients died while receiving active, aggressive cardiopulmonary resuscitation. For most patients, death was permitted only after a brutal and hard-nosed attempt to stave off the inevitable. Over time, the general practice of critical care mercifully evolved, and by the 1990s, most patients passed away in intensive care units without undergoing the anachronistic, vain ritual of cardiopulmonary resuscitation [4].

Countless hours were spent performing futile cardiopulmonary resuscitation on moribund patients whose lives were going to end notwithstanding any such heroic and well-intended interventions. I started to feel increasingly bitter and sarcastic regarding these useless interventions, which seemingly served no other purpose than to appease the sensibilities of other physicians and assuage the fears, anger, and hostility of otherwise unprepared patients and their families. Gradually, I questioned the morality of these interventions and increasingly permitted myself to interpose personal judgment concerning other's quality of life.

"What is the purpose of spending the entire night resuscitating this cancer-ridden nonagenarian, backside flayed to the bone with decubitus ulcers? There is no quality to her life. She lives dressed in diapers, unaware, bedridden in a nursing facility." These were the very darkest moments of my professional career.

I had the good fortune to read Robert Lifton's masterpiece, *The Nazi Doctors: Medical Killing and the Psychology of Genocide*, which helped prevent a continued slide down this dangerous moral slope of judging others' quality of life [5]. The phrase "lebensunwertes leben," or "life unworthy of life," the social and political underpinning of this grotesque nightmare, was chilling. I felt a growing sense of discomfiture regarding ruminations and judgments of patients' quality of life with the knowledge that willing collaboration of physicians was essential to purging society of those with "life unworthy of life."

The phrase, "life unworthy of life," struck a deep resonant chord, changed my attitude, and recalibrated my thinking. I would never again allow my personal perception of an acceptable quality of life influence decision-making concerning the propriety of a patient's life or death. Even so, the balance to remain neutral is difficult, and I continue to experience existential nausea and a sense of hopelessness resulting from the quotidian struggle regarding the unrealistic expectations of irresponsible physicians, hopelessly ill patients, and their devastated loved ones.

The Study to Understand Prognoses and Preferences for Outcomes and Risks of Treatments or SUPPORT served to reinforce the conclusions I had formulated from my own personal clinical experiences [6].

"The phase I observation documented shortcomings in communication, frequency of aggressive treatment, and the characteristics of hospital death: only 47 % of physicians knew when their patients preferred to avoid CPR; 46 % of do-not-resuscitate (DNR) orders were written within 2 days of death; 38 % of patients who died spent at least 10 days in an intensive care unit (ICU); and for 50 % of conscious patients who died in the hospital, family members reported moderate to severe pain at least half the time. During the phase II intervention, patients experienced no improvement in patient-physician communication (e.g., 37 % of control patients and 40 % of intervention patients discussed CPR preferences) or in the five targeted outcomes, i.e., incidence or timing of written DNR orders."

The perspective of this new mind-set motivated me to find effective strategies to cope with the unrelenting anguish engendered by the never-ending flow of unsalvageable patients into the intensive care unit. In numerous ways, the steadfast struggle to salvage those who can be saved with reasonable and measured means is less taxing than efforts to avoid dysthanasia and the orchestration of death with peace, comfort, and dignity. The decision to add a vasopressor, change an antibiotic, or make a ventilator change is made in a relatively brief moment compared to time needed to meet with families, discuss prognosis, establish milestones, and generate the bonds of trust needed to overcome fear, distrust, denial, and hostility. Though extremely gratifying, the emotional and psychological toll extracted by these more social activities has been extraordinarily wearing.

The practical reality is that many of the ethical crises encountered in the daily practice of critical care medicine can only be averted by a proactive and humane approach toward end-of-life planning prior to intensive care unit admission. My practice became more focused on preemptive efforts to forego vain heroics at the end of life. By necessity, I became involved in palliative care programs and initiatives and served not only as chief of critical care medicine but also helped develop and administrate several hospital-based palliative care services.

A singular travail with a very religious family still weighs heavily on my mind. Their loved one was dying of disseminated, metastatic lung cancer and was enduring a life of dependency, misery, and pain. He remained full code in the ICU, slowly dying on a mechanical ventilator with pneumonia. The family was adamant that he was to be resuscitated at all costs. Further, they enjoined me not to offer sedation or analgesia. In their opinion, the way to Heaven was to recapitulate the suffering of martyrdom on a cross. They believed that God had blessed me with medical skills and my duty was to use them to keep their loved alive, while his suffering served to ensure eternal joy in the afterlife. Every day for weeks on end, until he died, I negotiated, entreated, and argued with them for every milligram of morphine. Years later, I still remain haunted by images of his agonized facial contortions, as tearful nurses plead with resolute family members to stand aside so they could administer morphine. Would he have declined morphine if lucid? Did I interpose my personal quality of life perception while disrespecting his? Did I prevent him from dying in pain as perhaps he may have wanted and was he thus banished from Heaven? The ordeal of being enjoined to honor this request to prolong life with the specific intent of protracting suffering and the grueling struggle to offer appropriate analgesia notwithstanding the hostile, menacing, and scathing comments and glares still trouble me to this day.

The struggles I have with the specter of retirement are not grounded upon a real or perceived decline in mental or intellectual ability nor on a contrived notion indispensability. My psychological mind-set is such that I harbor no notion that work defines my personal worth. Whereas approximately one half of critical care physicians suffer from burnout, I do not suffer this syndrome in the classic sense as defined by Maslach [7, 8]. I do not feel depersonalized and harbor a sense of pride in my professional accomplishments. I do not suffer compassion fatigue, rather a colossal sense of moral fatigue, and profound disappointment concerning the dispassionate way medicine is all too often practiced.

The manner in which dying people are misled, mistreated, and abused is unconscionable. The failure to communicate openly and honestly and the specters of false hope, all exponentially enabled by dysfunctional fee-for-service reimbursement, are too often laid at the feet of the intensivist. For years, I have struggled with the misery and despair engendered by this perfect storm of neglect at the penultimate moment of thousands of lives. Desperate people are often encouraged to partake in grotesque medical misadventures, not truly informed nor cognizant of the horrific downside price to be extracted.

For example, terminally ill cancer patients receiving palliative chemotherapy suffer higher rates of cardiopulmonary resuscitation, mechanical ventilation, and late referrals to hospice, are more apt to expire in an intensive care unit, and are less likely to die at home or where they desire but with no increase in survival benefit [9]. In fact, palliative chemotherapy given to patients with end-stage cancer does not improve the experience of dying for those with moderate or poor performance status and degrades the experience of dying for patients who are performing reasonably well at baseline [10]. Further, it is known that earlier referrals for palliative care and the decision to forego aggressive care at the end of life are associated with not only a better quality of life but also longer survival [11]. Despite robust evidence that less aggressive care yields enhanced outcomes and a better death for many moribund patients, many physicians still demur and fail to have open, frank conversations with dying patients. All too often, intensivists must pick up the pieces of shattered expectations, and inevitably, over time, we pay an enormous emotional toll.

While helping a critically ill patient survive and return to an acceptable quality of life is extremely gratifying, facilitating a fellow man to die a peaceful, comfortable, and dignified death is equally very fulfilling. Further, assisting the loved ones of a terminally ill patient cope, find peace, and move forward is also extremely rewarding. In her book, *On Death and Dying*, Dr. Kübler-Ross elegantly delineates the psychological stages dying patients pass through [12]. Denial and isolation, anger, bargaining, depression, and final acceptance are experienced not only by the dying but also by their loved ones. I have come to realize that most conflict at the end of life is rooted in the asynchronous manner in which patients and their loved ones experience this final journey. From a practical sense, denial and anger are only natural when the patient's family first comes to learn of their loved one's disseminated, metastatic cancer from the intensivist. However wearing, it has been an honor, privilege, and very gratifying to work with even the most distressed and hostile families as they come to terms with the imminent and unexpected death of a loved one. The most satisfying moments often come after a patient and I have accepted the inevitable, and subsequently, we work together to harmonize a dysfunctional family into the phase of final acceptance and peace.

For me, the personal journey toward retirement is somewhat akin to phases of death and dying. At first, there was denial concerning the necessity or inevitability of retirement. Anger followed at the thought that so much might be left undone: with so many more lives to save, families to help, nurses and other coworkers to support, learners to teach, questions to answer, and systems to improve.

I have bargained with myself and others on many occasions and struck many deals. "I will feel better about phasing out once we have the recruited the requisite number faculty; will slow down once the protocols are finished and implemented; when the paper the fellow has been trying to publish is accepted; but until then, until then, until then…"

At present, I am emerging from depression associated with feelings of hopelessness and frustration regarding our dysfunctional healthcare system. I now begrudgingly accept that significant change will be slow and will not occur during the remainder of my professional lifetime. Patients will continue to be devastated by preventable illness and their families' lives torn apart. Physicians will continue to avoid difficult conversations with patients, who will tragically learn of the bleakness of their medical conditions only when faced with death in the intensive care unit. The social engineering required to recalibrate this dysfunction is the prime challenge of generations to come.

I have entered the stage of final acceptance regarding retirement from the practice of critical care medicine I have enjoyed for more than three decades and am at peace. I have accomplished much and have seen much accomplishment. No longer acrimonious, I have let go of my professional frustrations and simply wish to help pass the baton along to the next generation of critical care providers. I take great pride in the fact that my son has decided to follow in my footsteps and is about to embark on his own career in this wonderfully rewarding field of critical care medicine.

For the moment, I will continue to work at the bedside, to teach and mentor while arranging an orderly transition to the next generation of providers. The inexorable cycle of life has stationed me as mentor and advisor for many, and though not keen at the specter of my retirement, they will nonetheless do well when I step down and aside. The question of when I will finally lay down my stethoscope for the last time is not yet answered. However, one thing is clear: I have no intention of becoming yet another dispensable body in the graveyard of self-styled indispensable men.

My wife and best friend has persuaded me that I deserve some private time for peace and reflection. She has been at my side through extremely trying times and exhilarating moments. Many patients, their families, and I owe her an enormous debt of gratitude for keeping me even keeled through the worst moments of desolation and despair. The moment has come to repay that debt by offering her and our family the most precious gift of all, that of time together.

References

1. In the Matter of Karen Quinlan, an Alleged Incompetent. 70 N.J. 10 (1976) 355 A.2d 647.
2. Cruzan v. Director, Missouri Department of Health. 110 S. Ct. 2841 (1990).
3. Patient Self-Determination Act of 1990. H.R. 4449.
4. Prendergast TJ, Claessens MT, Luce JM. A national survey of end-of-life care for critically ill patients. Am J Respir Crit Care Med. 1998;158:1163–7.
5. Lifton RJ. The Nazi Doctors: medical killing and the psychology of genocide. ISBN 0-465-09094. 1986.
6. The SUPPORT Principal Investigators. A controlled trial to improve care for seriously ill hospitalized patients. The study to understand prognoses and preferences for outcomes and risks of treatments (SUPPORT). JAMA. 1995;274(20):1591–8.
7. Embriaco N, Azoulay E, Barrau K, Kentish N, Pochard F, Loundou A, Papazian L. High level of Burnout in intensivists prevalence and associated factors. Am J Respir Crit Care Med. 2007;175:686–92.
8. Maslach C. Burnout: the cost of caring. Englewood Cliffs: Prentice Hall; 1982.

9. Wright A, Zhang B, Keating N, Weeks J, Prigerson H. Associations between palliative chemotherapy and adult cancer patients' end of life care and place of death: prospective cohort study. BMJ. 2014;348:1219. doi:10.1136/bmj.g1219 (Published 4 March 2014).
10. Prigerson H, Bao Y, Shah MA, Paulk ME, LeBlanc TW, Schneider BJ, Garrido MM, Reid MC, Berlin DA, Adelson KB, Neugut AI, Maciejewski PK. Chemotherapy use, performance status, and quality of life at the end of life. JAMA Oncol. 2015;1(6):778–84. doi:10.1001/jamaoncol.2015.2378.
11. Temel JS, Greer JA, Muzikansky A, Gallagher ER, Admane S, Jackson VA, Dahlin CM, Blinderman CD, Jacobsen J, Pirl WF, Billings JA, Lynch TJ. Early palliative care for patients with metastatic non–small-cell lung cancer. NEJM. 2010;363:733–42.
12. Ross K-R. On death and dying. What the dying have to teach doctors, nurses, clergy, and their own families. ISBN 978-1-4767-7554-8. 1969.

Chapter 13
The Ageing Intensivist and Functional Incapacity

Brad Power

Introduction

I was in danger of losing my 'quiz night team', smart nerd position. Something was taking names from my brain. Minutiae like naming the irritating kid in a 1960s TV program could disappear. I would enthusiastically think 'I know that one' but then not be able to name him. It might be back the next day. I was 52.

Our hospital pharmacology professor told me of an intern he trained with at Sydney University, named George. George produced a low-budget 2 or 3 minute film to open the Sydney Hospital comedy revue. A movie screen and opening film reveal a vaguely identifiable figure standing distantly on Sydney Harbour entrance cliffs, holding a statue of Liberty flame. A plane (George had persuaded someone to fund it) approaches over ocean. It steadily targets 'Liberty'. Liberty Lady falls unglamorously to the ground. As she falls, her face reveals her to be the dour aged female pathologist from the pathology laboratory. She was legendary to all, named on pathology report slips, but it was reputed never to have emerged in daylight. George Miller did 1 year as an intern doctor in Sydney. He then directed the initial 1981 Mad Max movie (USA, 'Road Warrior') and its famous follow-up movies. George's latest film has just won 6 Oscars. Mad Max films led Mel Gibson to fame.

I hate Mel Gibson. I'm sure he was involved in closing down my medical career. I'll come back to this.

I like my neurologist. He has cared for me since 2009 (age 52), although his opening words on consultation of 'Brad, this is bad' were disturbing. I'll come back to this.

B. Power, MD
Senior Intensive Care Specialist, Department of Intensive Care,
Sir Charles Gairdner Hospital, Perth, Western Australia, Australia
e-mail: bradicu@iinet.net.au

© Springer International Publishing Switzerland 2016
D. Crippen (ed.), *The Intensivist's Challenge: Aging and Career Growth in a High-Stress Medical Specialty*, DOI 10.1007/978-3-319-30454-0_13

Getting to Medicine

My mother said to me in 1974 when I was 17, 'University is free again; it won't last long…make use of it'. My mother's free education in 1942–1946 at the University of Western Australia (UWA), the first free university in the British Empire, had allowed her to gain a degree in Mathematics and Biochemistry. Women born in 1923 in Australia had usually not been able to afford and had not been encouraged to get university education. She valued education. Employment did not even necessarily follow for women at the end of World War II, and thus she spent much of her adult life raising children. Growing wealth in Australia in the mid-1960s and 1970s allowed some professional women to return to the workforce. My older sister was still advised in 1969 that careers for smart women were still confined to teaching, banking or nursing, to be ceased upon marriage.

The social change of the mid-1970s Australia saw a multi-gender and broader social group enter into medicine and made it very vibrant and enjoyable. About a third of our year class were women. I had good university training and was fortunate to be one of the two Honour Graduates out of 100 in our year of medicine. The other was an awesome graduate and she was the state's Rhodes Scholar. My sporting prowess was limited to 'Pinball'.

I had enjoyed every day at high school. I enjoyed every day at the university. On employment entry, I loved clinical work. I have loved teaching and the exposure it has given me to future generations. I have loved working in the sociable environment of hospitals and specifically in critical care specialities. I have loved being able to care for patients and their families. At age 59 I think I am not old.

Research was not my strong suit. Dr Barry Marshall, my first medical registrar, asked in the mid-1980s would I like to help on his project with *Campylobacter pylori* (later *Helicobacter pylori*). I think my reply was something like, 'Barry, that will come to nothing…I am going to do some ICU research into Bioimpedance measurement of cardiac output'. I was ahead of my time? Barry has a Nobel Prize.

Picking the wind of change was also never my strong suit. During my Physician Fellowship study in 1983 or 1984, I'm pretty sure I said (loudly) 'Why should we subscribe to The New England Journal of Medicine when all it publishes is stuff on some odd disease in gay men in San Francisco and how can anything ever come from that!' I missed the first case of HIV I saw then, and indeed I think the first likely case of this illness in Australia was thus missed by me.

Mel Gibson

At age 52, I was on a 4-h flight from Perth to Sydney to attend a medical conference. I reflected on my first flight to Sydney some 30 years before to attend a student medical conference. I had enjoyed the movie 'Tim (Warner Brothers)' [1] on that earlier flight. As I reminisced, I realised that I could 'see' Mel Gibson's face, but I could not 'name' him. I could visualise him in Mad Max 1 (USA, Road Warrior) [2] with its odd characters and Mad Max 2 and indeed all of his movies and their suppporting cast, but I couldn't pull Mel's name. Gone, totally gone. I probably worked it out after going through the alphabet letter by letter a few times.

If I was to meet Mel, I would have just had to have stuck out my paw and hoped that he introduced himself or that his name would have come. I *could* remember Piper Laurie who was in Tim. Piper was fantastic. I think if we'd met she'd have liked me, although in her autobiography [3], I could see that she wasn't keen on Ronald Reagan. I could remember Colleen McCulloch who had written the book *Tim*. She had written the book whilst working as a neuroscientist at Yale. Now there was a strong medical link. Whilst Mel's name has disappeared somewhere from the naming centre in my brain, my brain's minutiae centre where useless facts reside, was working overtime.

Colleen McCullough died in early 2015, only months before I started this publication. In 1978, the professor of medicine at the Royal Perth Hospital (an Indian cardiologist, previously one of Idi Amin's physicians in Uganda, not a job conducive to longevity) had invited our medical student group to lunch. He was dining with a 'person who might interest us'. Not knowing who Colleen McCullough was, but aware that it was not a name we associated with any large Australian brewer, my group maintained its plan for our end-of-week drinking session. She'd just written *The Thorn Birds* [4].

Interestingly, Colleen's training as a doctor was stopped by soap allergy, leading her to a career in laboratory neuroscience. She had established a neurophysiology clinic at the Royal North Shore Hospital in Sydney (I'll ask Malcolm Fisher about that) and worked at the Great Ormond Street Hospital in the UK and Yale in the USA. She has said that she wrote *Tim* and *The Thorn Birds* during her 10 years at Yale to supplement her low income. Had she been a US neurosurgeon, perhaps a two-million dollar grossing book would just have been accounted for in the petty cash.

McCullough was more memorable to me for the fact that Richard Chamberlain had the lead role as Father Ralph in *The Thorn Birds* TV miniseries. Now Richard Chamberlain was the irrepressible 'Dr Kildare' and what doctors were meant to be like. Not a Ben Casey, not a Dr Zorba nor even Marcus Welby, but he was pretty good. I do believe that a few questions on Ben Casey or Dr Zorba in my physician or later ICU exams might have allowed recognition that my education was broader than that of some 'nerdy' students who had spent too much time studying. Sadly that never occurred. Nevertheless I occasionally did slip questions into bedside rounds, about Vince Edwards or Sam Jaffe or even 'Doc' from *Combat* (he had no second name) to identify Fellows who I thought showed appreciation of medicine's finer points.

The Neurologist

It's time to go mention the neurologist. We had trained together. I bumped into him in a hospital car park. I was returning (it was night) to the hospital, he was just leaving (neurologist clinics always run hours late). If I hadn't run into him, I probably would just have stalled further making an appointment. Like most issues relating to doctors and personal health, that seemed a good spot to explain my 'minor concern'.

I stated that I felt I had 'lost' some names. I outlined the Mel Gibson conspiracy. I really had noted similar problems of slowness with names on other occasions and all that was missing 'was the name'. I had dealt with it by just going methodically through the alphabet. Sometimes they just 'came' during this process or I would 'clear' the 'waiting to send names' as I relaxed in bed at night. It was not frequent but I knew it was not right.

I knew enough neurology to be worried about my dominant temporal lobe. Medical specialists have to use 'words' a lot and so my warning sign was early. I described the absence of other temporal lobe phenomena such as *deja vu* or *jamais vu*. Twice in my career, my patient had been diagnosed with temporal lobe tumours, manifesting as having experienced odd smells or tastes. One having a seizure after taking his wife's cooking off the stove and throwing out the door 'cos it stank'; a second admitted to the hospital for investigation whereupon he suddenly started running along the corridor yelling 'fire...fire' from the olfactory hallucinations. In assessing suspected encephalitis, I would remind registrars of the above, not to mention George Gershwin who whilst playing Rhapsody in Blue on stage, paused and was blank for some seconds before resuming. Questioned later, he said he smelled burning rubber. He presented to a hospital only weeks later 'coning' from his brain tumour. I would tell fellows of a young lady who had developed Klüver-Bucy syndrome complicating delayed diagnosis of herpes encephalitis, sadly leaving her totally sexually inappropriate. I didn't have that problem.

I told him that I always remembered that as a child aged ten, my school teacher had shown me some dictation that had been handed in, and there were five or six lines of 'purely disconnected garble'. I made the mistake of laughing (teacher's pet) and asking 'who wrote that' and he responded ... 'you'. I'd always wondered if it was a childhood seizure. I was only ever concussed once (university orientation party), and I was the least likely candidate for sports-related chronic traumatic encephalopathy.

In retrospect I did have some other mild things. I was increasingly tired by day. I thought that faces 'looked funny' but couldn't describe how. As a separate feature and on reflection, my ability to play George's Rhapsody in Blue without the sheet music had probably been lost over some months.

The neurologist told me to have an MRI and come and see him. The mailed request was for a cerebral MRI with D2-weighted imaging.

An opening comment of 'Brad this is Bad', with a bit of a stare, prompted my considered response of 'Mmmmm, I know'. A lengthier pause was followed by a 'Brad, this is really bad'. Communication is my strong suit, and I thought at the time.... 'This is probably bad!' My neurology skills had not been too bad because my dominant temporal lobe MRI images did have a lot of 'black dots' in them which he indicated were deposits of haemosiderin, the black dot appearance making them look like 'holes'. What I had not appreciated was that there would also be a huge number of very small black spots in many many areas of my brain. It had more 'holes' than after the Al Capone St. Valentine's Day Massacre.

I appreciated the expertise of my neurologist. The hemosiderin was from small vessel bleeds of varying ages. The vessel abnormality was due to amyloid deposition within the blood vessel walls making them brittle. It fell under the classification of a 'cerebral micro-haemorrhage syndrome'. The distribution and nature of bleeds were virtually diagnostic of cerebral amyloid angiopathy (CAA). [5] He had an excellent understanding and experience on cerebral amyloid angiopathy including caring for a family of patients with familial CAA. I was unfortunate to have it occur at my age. He guessed that as the only Spanish I could recite to him was 'dos cervezas por favor' I was unlikely Mexican, and moved the differential diagnosis of multiple cavernous angiomas down his list. He didn't need many tests save to exclude a few rare things. I was not Icelandic or Dutch.

My first lecture in Pathology at UWA was inflammation (useful for my ICU work), the second was Amyloid. It was the lead question in my final pathology examination. I won the prize for the subject. I thought of my mnemonic for the Type 1 amyloid accumulated muscle site of Skeletal, Heart, Intestine and Tongue. I had seen unusual clinical presentations during my clinical career and thought of the lady who had presented with a massive tongue, leading to our trial of an industrial solvent DMSO. Hers was a different amyloid syndrome and I hoped I would not end up smelling like new furniture. I always knew amyloid would get some payback on me! This was an unusual form of amyloid confined to affecting cerebral blood vessels.

On the way home after the consultation, my partner had perhaps over-optimistically moved the 'decimal point of the likelihood of good times calculation', to the right of mine. I was less sanguine. I reduced my commentary to 'This is pretty bad'. I think the friendly qualifier 'pretty' was about as supportive as I could be that night. I was also considering whether it was appropriate to still buy green bananas.

Coming Out

My wife is a barrister. I learned one of my most useful concepts for practicing medicine when we had first met. She had said 'Do you know where I start when I get given a new brief…?' The ultimate answer turned out to be 'I imagine I am giving my final address to the judge. It is to get to the best available outcome for my client. Every step in getting to that point is logical, goal focused and strategic'. She recounted how some clients came along having trawled the Internet and thought they had found some point which nobody else had realised was important. They consequently made bad decisions, their outcomes were worse and more costly. I glibly thought, 'Gee I've seen lots of patients and families like that'.

She then said that often opposing lawyers 'Lost sight of the big picture and run arguments which may have seem clever but were of no value'. They ran arguments which were not going to succeed, they sought injunctions which delayed resolution and they did not help their client, costing them only money and pain. I remembered more solemnly thinking, 'Gee I see a lot of doctors doing that, doing things just because they can but with no strategic advantage for their patient'. Stephen Streat has used the term SODs (Single Organ Doctors) for this sort of medical approach.

So what did I do?

1. Many of my plans for patients 'start at the end' of what is the best outcome I can get for them. It seemed logical that I should apply the same philosophy to myself. I knew at some stage that I would need to stop working. I could not beat the odds. I accepted that; the question then was what was important to me and

how would I get there. I was a bedside tertiary level intensive care specialist. That's what I wanted to do whilst I could. It was the best thing I had done in my life. I wanted to do it as I had always done, working hard and spending time at the bedside, spending time mentoring doctors in training and time supporting patients and their families. I wanted to keep doing my 'share of the work' and that included a significant number of after-hours shifts. Of importance, I did not want to be remembered as the person who did not know when to go. I did not want to be remembered as someone who became dangerous. I did not wish my biography to become a sad one of someone who made stupid mistakes by ignoring the obvious. My job as a role model was to show to others that 'when it's time to go, it's time to go'. At the time of diagnosis, my function was well preserved, and although I was aware of some word-finding difficulties and 'what was different', my colleagues were not.

2. Since approximately 2010, medical practitioners caring for doctors in Australia with 'impairment' have had a mandatory requirement to notify medical registration bodies. 'Impairment' is difficult to define but is taken as when illness has caused disability sufficient to be a threat to patient care. All states in Australia require reporting of various at risk behaviours, and all require doctors to report 'impaired' doctors who they are treating even if they may have a plan which is seemingly working. My state of Western Australia is the only state to exempt treating practitioners from the need to make such reports [6]. It is argued that obligatory reporting especially in the case where a treatment plan has been formed will decrease the likelihood that such practitioners will seek care. Readers may wish to consider the legislation in their state or country when they realise a colleague has become impaired. Separately, what do you do with respect to an impaired colleague, when you are the treating doctor? It should be noted that notifications for organic brain injury like mine are actually uncommon, and most 'impairment to practise' is due to psychiatric illness (often being well managed and controlled) and drug abuse. Notwithstanding, I found myself with an illness, not necessarily 'impaired' at first instance, but also in a situation where should I deteriorate my treating clinician was not bound to report me to the medical board.

3. What did I do? Intensive care medicine can be a 'ticking bomb' in terms of a patient experiencing a bad outcome with the immediate conclusion that 'the doctor must have done something wrong'. Notification of an independent regulatory body, determination of any practice restrictions and, working within those professional limits is perhaps your best protection. It is useful to know that this is a standard you expect from your entire department and institutional colleagues, for the protection of them, you and your institution.

I notified my practice colleagues and gave them tacit approval to notify the medical registration board should they have any concern. I did not want to compromise them. I told my wife that I wished her to report me should she have any concern about my cognition or behaviour. My wife had been a member of the Legal Practice Tribunal and was aware of management of 'Impaired Colleagues'. I did not want to compromise her. I notified my employer. Despite the absence of a regulation to notify regulatory bodies, I voluntarily notified the Medical Registration Board and supplied full details of my illness and supplied all reports and scans. I gave them written approval to contact my colleagues and my wife as they felt necessary. I think she might have been a 'dobber' if I even blinked badly. Voluntary notification was accompanied by written permission to my clinician to allow all reporting requirements. I did not wish him to be conflicted by patient confidentiality. I did not seek to interfere with these reports. The medical board ensured that I kept employing bodies aware if any limits were to be placed but respected my privacy. It did not make reports available on websites. I had no regrets about following an open disclosure approach.

4. I was fortunate in the choices available to me in my post-diagnosis career. First I was not 'too' 'impaired' and the medical board took a 'watching role'. Second, medicine had been well rewarded in Australia and also I had good income protection. The country had enjoyed a golden age of wealth and social support in terms of leave. I was thus most fortunate in that finances were not a major driver of whether I chose to work or 'lifestyle refocus'. The reader may wish to consider the pressures which might encourage some to continue working even with a significant health problem. I have seen practitioners who have not carried appropriate life and income protection insurance.

5. Role models from my working career were a major guider of my actions. Prof. Malcolm Fisher had once opined at a meeting 'Being good at ICU involves working hard and doing the nights. When you can't do the nights, you're in trouble!' I had loved night work as part of my work. You see the other side of the hospital and of illness. I saw my job as to do the full mix. In 2014, at age 56, I decided that I could not or should not do the night work and I should cease. That had been my plan since diagnosis. That is what I did. Sad, but I had no regrets.

6. A role modelling renal physician who had been a legendary hospital consultant had once said to me 'When I retire, I am going out the door and I am not coming back. It's not that I have hated the hospital, rather the reverse. It's just that I know I need to have planned something else to do'. I might say that he did return 2 months later, and to the ICU, with a closed head injury when he fell off a ladder. Fortunately he recovered fully and he returns each year now to bestow the teaching award named after him. I do not climb ladders.

7. When I ceased 'clinical medicine', I thus ceased it completely and in a planned fashion. I sit on ethics committees at two large hospitals. I read medical literature. I read some fiction, but it takes a long time to recover that skill. My apartment overlooks my hospital of over 30 years, but I make few trips to it. We all remember the baseballer, the soccer player or the cricketer who stays on just that little bit too long. That is not the memory that I wish my colleagues to have.

8. I was fortunate in that my self-appreciated 'losses' were always going to be at a pace not necessarily appreciable to others but 'sad' and readily appreciable to me. This is compared with the slower changes of normal ageing. I could not live in the land of denial.

9. What did I notice during the 2 years after diagnosis? Functionally I could look OK if I tried. Most colleagues said they didn't realise much. But one's usual traits are accentuated. I found that I was more obsessive in things I did. I was always fatigued. I made sure I attended any night on-call work or emergencies. I knew it would be easy to just avoid that one episode where I would always

previously have gone in but I knew that going in had always made me safe. My documentation was more obsessive and my orders were more extensive. I had always enjoyed my words (I was always impressed by Stephen Streat and Rolando Berger and Steven Hollenberg who used words and ideas so deftly on CCM-L) and to lose words was my greatest sadness.

10. As I type the corrections to the proofs on this page the movie Mad Max Fury Road has just won 6 Academy awards. I think that bloke whose name I can't remember and who made me start this chapter, wasn't in it. I like George Miller though. I think he's a role model for a new career.

11. What's the most important thing I did? When I was diagnosed, my partner thought it was a good time to make me her husband. It seemed a good idea. It has been.

References

1. Tim 1979 Pisces Production. Adapted from the novel Tim by Colleen McCullough.
2. Mad Max 1979 Kennedy Miller Productions Village Roadshow Pictures.
3. Learning to Live out Loud A Memoir. Piper Laurie. Amazon Books 2011.
4. The Thorn Birds (1977) Colleen McCullough Harper and Rowe.
5. Yamada M (2015) Cerebral amyloid angiopathy: Emerging concepts. J Stroke 17(1): 17–30.
6. Goiran HN et al (2014) Mandatory reporting of health professionals: the case for a Western Australian style exemption for all Australian practitioners. J Law Med 22(1): 209–220.

Chapter 14
Legacy: What Ageing Intensivists Can Pass On

Stephen Streat

The Beginning

Critical care began early in my country. The first ICU in New Zealand [1] opened in late 1958 contemporaneously with other very early ICUs in the USA [2] and less than 6 years after what might be the beginning of what we now call intensive or critical care medicine [3–5]. That first New Zealand ICU was directed by Dr Matthew (Matt) Spence, a Glaswegian anaesthetist who emigrated in 1952 to work in what is now the Auckland City Hospital. He described himself in 1986 in an after-dinner speech at an Australian conference as "a cantankerous Scot…mellowed by 34 years in New Zealand", but this mellowing was less evident in 1974 when, as a final year medical student, I first met him in the alien sci-fi moonscape [6] of the ICU. By that time, 16 years after it opened, the ICU was still in an old converted infectious diseases ward built in the 1930s but had grown to employ three full-time specialists, all of whom had trained first in anaesthesia and who had brought many other skills to their ongoing exploration of what was even then largely an uncharted region of medical space.

At school I had always been an "outlier", what would later become known as a geek. In the 1960s I was interested in music, politics, the space programme and the new science of computing and in the 1970s in medicine (especially physiology and psychiatry) and what we now know as information and communication technology. In our final year as medical students, we could do a 3-month elective project in any hospital or university in which we could find an approved supervisor. In 1974, I chose "creative computing and cybernetics" in the School of Fine Arts and used a

S. Streat, FRACP
Department of Critical Care Medicine, Auckland City Hospital,
2 Park Road, Grafton, Auckland 1023, New Zealand

Organ Donation New Zealand, Newmarket, PO Box 99431, Auckland 1149, New Zealand
e-mail: Stephens@adhb.govt.nz

© Springer International Publishing Switzerland 2016
D. Crippen (ed.), *The Intensivist's Challenge: Aging and Career Growth in a High-Stress Medical Specialty*, DOI 10.1007/978-3-319-30454-0_14

DEC PDP8/e with laboratory peripherals in the Department of Psychiatry to dabble in "desktop" computing (a chess programme in 4 K of octal core, short 16 mm movies shot frame-by-frame from computed images, real-time animations in response to musical inputs and some interactive adjuncts to clinical decision-making).

Unsurprisingly perhaps, the ICU in the 1970s gave me the opportunity to pursue some of these personal interests, in a less constrained learning and working environment than the traditional hierarchical formality of medicine and surgery. The ICU was the "domain of freer spirits" and some arcane phenomenological concepts – "adult respiratory distress syndrome" [7], "multiple organ failure" [8], "acute brain swelling" [9] and "hypoxic-ischaemic encephalopathy" [10]. We used novel and creative combinations of physiological therapies to "support the patient" until time and a few specific treatments, mostly surgical, could facilitate healing and recovery. The ICU was a "citadel" with a close nursing and medical team. We relied on bedside clinical examination and observation. There was little physiological monitoring and few special investigations. Intuition, inductive reasoning and pattern recognition were highly valued skills which were often rewarded. Much later we came to realise how our diagnostic conclusions, treatments and outcomes were biased by the limitations of these methods, including confirmation bias. Most treatments were not evidence based in terms of a clinically meaningful end point (survival)! We used treatments which produced short-term "improvements" in physiology which we hoped or blithely assumed "should" or "would" lead to better outcomes for our patients. Although there were a few (e.g. [11]) very early randomised controlled trials in our speciality, most of our simple yet powerful treatments (e.g. mechanical ventilatory support, catecholamine infusion, blood volume expansion) were supported only by "uncontrolled cohort studies", "expert opinion" or "extrapolation from very short-duration animal studies".

I realised that many of my contemporaries did not like having to make life-and-death decisions under conditions of often considerable diagnostic uncertainty (no CT or MR scans, little point-of-care laboratory testing, limited bedside radiology, very simple ultrasound). I found that I could at least attempt this with reasonable equanimity. I saw how our simple intensive therapies could make a crucial difference to patient's survival and quality of life and appreciated the rich opportunity that the ICU gave me for learning and later for teaching.

After brief forays into psychiatry and what would soon become emergency medicine, I returned to the serious business of training in internal medicine which in Australian and New Zealand had just recognised intensive care medicine as a legitimate speciality. I think that like others of my contemporaries, I was "at the right place at the right time" and fell into intensive care medicine serendipitously, in part perhaps because no other speciality would have tolerated me, much less supported me.

The period of my formal training in intensive care medicine (1977–1982) was one of the great technological advancements and rapid changes. We saw ventilators become software driven, with their resultant peculiarities and strengths, the rise of invasive haemodynamic monitoring, ICP monitoring, point-of-care testing, safe and effective parenteral nutrition, purpose-built enteral feeds, safe and effective ICU haemodialysis, early internal fixation of fractures, permissive hypercarbia in ARDS, routine use of CT and bedside neurophysiology, ICU severity and scoring systems and audit, the beginning of ICU clinical research and many other aspects of the "invisible infrastructure" of the modern ICU.

I was fortunate to be asked to work as a surgical research fellow by the late Professor Graham Hill [12] who saw that having a physician intensivist in his team would extend his clinical research (e.g. 13–16) into the intensive care unit. However, this 3-year period of intense exposure to surgical patients, surgical thinking and surgical research taught me a great deal about patient care, including about the surgical covenantal ethic [17], the importance of therapeutic simplicity, good housekeeping, non-intervention and the passage of time as crucial aspects of survival in complex critical surgical illness. I was again serendipitously in the right place at the right time.

I returned to intensive care medicine as a full-time specialist in 1985. By this time, much of intensive care medicine had been somewhat systematised – particularly in the treatment of acute respiratory failure, shock, trauma, asthma, drug overdose but even in the more difficult problems of sepsis, traumatic brain injury and other cerebral catastrophes. Intensivists, including me, began to appreciate and acknowledge the limits of our therapeutic capabilities. Along with that appreciation, we became increasingly aware of the accompanying moral issues, including the potential preventability of many of the catastrophes we were called upon to treat, the human and fiscal calculus of resource allocation, what the French so eloquently call "acharnement thérapeutique", the dilemma of survival with tolerable or intolerable disability and the importance of compassion, sensitivity, patient- and family-centred care and communication [18]. We found it easier to acknowledge our own weaknesses, humanity, frailty and mortality.

The Course

Over the first 15 years or so of my clinical work as a specialist intensivist (1985–2000), there were quite a few highlights, and it's hard to see what in retrospect I would have done differently. Intensive care medicine as a speciality came of age in many ways – it developed and consolidated its own identity, including training, clinical practice, research, publication and collegiality. My professional practice, as part of a small close-knit group of intensivists, included busy clinical activities in the ICU along with both primary prevention [19] and what we now call rapid-response teams. Locally we worked hard and with long hours at the bedside, audited our practice using a prospective clinical database and developed our clinical practice. As a result of what we came to see as gaps in our practice, we began nurse-led follow-up services for bereaved relatives [18] and for ICU survivors shortly after hospital discharge [20] along with some outreach in-hospital activities. We embraced the Internet as a medium for communication and information exchange. Our geographic isolation in the South Pacific gives New Zealanders (a nation of world travellers) an appreciation of the power of the Internet to create a more level playing field in intensive care medicine, as well as many other aspects of international discourse and business. In 1994 I stumbled across a small black and white picture of David Crippen holding a stethoscope up to a computer screen in a newsletter to members of the Society of Critical Care Medicine. I was an early contributor to CCM-L and through this association made a large number of fine collegial contacts and some very close personal friends.

I am proud (and fortunate, I think) to have been part of the Australian and New Zealand practices of intensive care medicine. Intensivists in our two countries have worked closely together since the original meetings in the early 1970s between the small number of intensive care practitioners who were both pioneers and friends [21]. The Australian and New Zealand Intensive Care Society (ANZICS) was formed in 1975 and elected Dr Matthew (Matt) Spence as the first president and Dr Robert (Bob) Wright, from Sydney, as secretary. The Society held its first Annual Scientific Meeting in Melbourne in 1975 and its fortieth in Auckland in October 2015.

ANZICS is a vibrant and active professional society which sees itself "advocate for intensive care throughout Australia and New Zealand" and which is "…devoted to all aspects of intensive care medical practice through ongoing professional education, the provision of leadership in medical settings, clinical research and analysis of critical care resources". The ANZICS Clinical Trials Group (ANZICS-CTG), founded in 1994, figures prominently in intensive care research (e.g. 22–25) and provides another opportunity for strong binational collegial linkages, engagement and career satisfaction. This Australian and New Zealand consortium now includes 70 ICUs, has over 180 publications in peer-reviewed journals and continues to grow in capability, funding, activity and research outcomes. As someone who supports the CTG and works in an ICU which contributes strongly to CTG-endorsed research, I see how involvement in clinical research is a powerful legacy tool. Clinical ICU research is best conducted in units with a good "housekeeping" infrastructure wherein unwarranted clinical practice variation is minimised, and there are standard approaches to all of the "routine" aspects of intensive care medicine. It is often said that standardised care itself (including participation in trials with standardised protocols) may improve outcome and there is some evidence to support this [26, 27]. Standardisation improves the "signal to noise ratio" of interventional studies [28] and so emphasises the clinical value of such a style of practice to other members of the ICU team. Participation in clinical research has, in my experience, a positive effect upon the degree of engagement of staff in an academic knowledge of the topic under study and also upon wider issues concerning research design, informed consent, performance of trials, analysis and presentation of results and applicability of published research to one's own clinical setting.

I saw the benefits to my Australian ICU colleagues in Sydney and Brisbane that liver transplantation had in the late 1980s and became heavily involved in the establishment of a single national liver transplant service in New Zealand in the late 1990s. This successful service [29–31] has had a substantial flow-on effect for non-transplant patients with liver disease as well as for the ICU and the hospital that provide the service.

The Evolution

I have always had an interest in both transplantation and organ donation. In the late 1970s in both nephrology and ICU, I treated renal transplant patients and discussed organ donation with the families of potential donors in the ICU. When New Zealand began a national heart transplant programme 10 years later, I had assisted the establishment of a national organ donation coordination office. An opportunity arose in 2005 to work part-time in this field as a (medical) director of what is now our national organ donation agency ("Organ Donation New Zealand"). At the same time, I was asked to participate in a novel activity for me – hospital-based health technology assessment [32] as deputy chair of a clinical practice committee. We were charged with assessing the safety, efficacy and cost utility of proposed new treatments or services and advising hospital management about their prioritisation and implementation. While working as a liver transplant surgeon at the Mayo Clinic in Minnesota, the chair of this committee had seen the value that such an approach can bring to an organisation and succeeded in establishing such a committee in Auckland. This committee has expanded over time and now advises four publically funded health service providers (serving ~2 million people in four contiguous regions). As a result I began to work in two places – alternating weekly between organ donation and health technology assessment and clinical work in the ICU.

I realised how easy it is to get overextended. I also realised how working in multiple departments ran the risk that each department could think that their particular priorities on time were (slightly) more important than other department priorities. Many of my intensivist colleagues now work in multiple (non-ICU) roles and experience similar pressures. Some of these roles are more "traditional", e.g. anaesthesia, but others are involved in senior positions of medical governance or leadership – in a variety of non-ICU fields including prehospital emergency care, government, quality assurance, teaching, research and hospital administration.

The multidisciplinary nature of ICU practice requires intensivists to have a broad if basic understanding of other clinical disciplines and some facility "speaking everyone's languages". Being a good intensivist also requires a disciplined approach to assessing risks, benefits and cost utility and the ability to creatively "problem-solve" in complex situations, including ones for which there is no "existing pathway". Good intensivists can talk about and help with "difficult" human matters – such as death and dying (including loss, grief and bereavement), patient's choices and preferences, making decisions under conditions of uncertainty and all of the emotions and behaviours that accompany these matters. These intensivist "life skills" are highly transferable to other non-ICU areas, and intensivists should feel confident that there are other opportunities to add value to other workplaces, as an alternative to "the ICU call roster" – especially when age is advancing and it takes longer to bounce back from the rigours of night work and irregular sleep.

Burnout [33] ("… physical, emotional and mental exhaustion from one's job or career") is a problem for intensivists, although perhaps not as prevalent in ICU as it is in emergency medicine or psychiatry. Increasing work-related stress without an accompanying increase in work satisfaction has been highlighted as impacting the mental health of senior doctors and intensivists must pay attention to managing that work-related stress (including by personal strategies and by advocating for their working conditions) as well as continuing to find personal satisfaction in the work – which might come in various ways for different individuals. Having a long, healthy and productive career in intensive care medicine requires each individual to find their appropriate balance between stress and satisfaction and pay attention to maintaining that balance in the face of the inevitability of ongoing change in the working environment. As a personal example, I have found that working as a member of a number of expert committees (e.g. those responsible for the ANZICS Statements on Death and Organ Donation and on Care at the End of Life [34, 35]) has increased my job satisfaction despite the additional work-related stress!

Intensivists in particular see daily evidence of the fragile and unpredictable nature of the human condition. Critical illness often occurs suddenly and without warning. Patients often die in the ICU within a few days of illness, and these deaths can often strike us as premature or even cruel. Daily we are confronted by death and by new-onset disability. We see other life-threatening conditions (diabetes, heart disease, cancer, degenerative neurological conditions) increasingly occurring in ourselves and our peers as we age. I like to think that we use this experience to develop our compassion and sensitivity, rather than increasing our fear of death and disability. I hope that it enhances our ability to support and help our patients and their families to also face these issues, "squarely and with fortitude".

I was asked to consider the specific issue of "legacy" – from the perspective of the "ageing intensivist". As many colleagues much older than me are heard to say "I don't feel like an ageing intensivist" but the number of years "on the clock" forces me to accept this description. I wryly smile when the junior staff refer to patients in their 60s or 70s as "this old chap". I most keenly feel like a "stranger in a strange land" when I vividly recount game-changing clinical events or publications of 30 or 40 years ago, and the junior staff tell me that this was in "prehistory" (being a time well before most of them were born, let alone had any interest in such matters).

It is naïve and vain to think that our legacy will be momentous or durable or that our moral worth should be measured by our tangible legacy. I know that my legacy, like that of most humans, will be transient and soon forgotten. We are remembered by those whose lives we have touched and by those who hear about their stories of us. Our patients and their families remember us as "people", more for the way we have treated them with honesty, compassion, understanding and some sharing of our own humanity and less as "doctors" or by whether we were technically proficient or clever in the way that we provided treatments or developed clinical services or activities. Some of us have been privileged to have contributed more generally to the evolving jigsaw of medical knowledge that we now refer to anachronistically as "the literature", and all of us have been "clinical teachers" in some way – at the bedside, in the hospital or university and to a variety of healthcare colleagues. We know that most clinical knowledge has a "half-life" of less than a decade and that any contribution we made to discovery is likely to be part of an interesting hospital footnote in a generation (or two). Knowledge and "truth" in our speciality has changed enormously in its 60-year lifespan so far, contrasting starkly with the durability of Einstein's general theory of relativity, still holding up well and published exactly a century ago.

Generation Passing

I began my specialist practice in the early 1980s, watching the "first generation" of intensivists, my seniors by 20 years or more, who were grappling with mid- and late-career options, legacy and retirement for the first time in intensive care medicine. I owe them an enormous debt for their "shoulders that I stood on" as well as for their openness and generosity in teaching me most of what I know about these more ephemeral but defining aspects of intensive care medicine. Some of our "pioneers" worked up to a retirement date and simply stopped, never to enter the hospital again. Others worked part-time in intensive care and increasingly took up other interests, both medical and non-medical, before finally retiring from clinical medicine in their 70s but continuing to remain connected and involved with the intensive care medicine in various ways. We are now defining these pathways for ourselves, and I think that we can give heart to our successors that there will be a satisfying pathway which is best for each of us. We should not fret about legacy and have no need to "rage, rage against the dying of the light". Personally I hope to continue to be able to make choices from a menu of work possibilities that allows me to contribute, as long as I want to, as long as I can and as long as that contribution is wanted and of value.

References

1. Spence M. The emergency treatment of acute respiratory failure. Anesthesiology. 1962;23:524–37.
2. Safar P, Dekornfeld TJ, Pearson JW, Redding JS. The intensive care unit. A three year experience at Baltimore city hospitals. Anaesthesia. 1961;16:275–84.
3. Trubuhovich RV. August 26th 1952 at Copenhagen: 'Bjørn Ibsen's Day'; a significant event for Anaesthesia. Acta Anaesthesiol Scand. 2004;48(3):272–7.
4. Lassen HCA. Preliminary report on the 1952 epidemic of poliomyelitis in Copenhagen with special reference to the treatment of acute respiratory insufficiency. Lancet. 1953;1:37–41.
5. Berthelsen PG, Cronqvist M. The first intensive care unit in the world: Copenhagen 1953. Acta Anaesthesiol Scand. 2003;47:1190–5.
6. Cassell J. Life and death in intensive care. Philadelphia: Temple University Press; 2005.
7. Ashbaugh DG, Bigelow DB, Petty TL, Levine BE. Acute respiratory distress in adults. Lancet. 1967;2(7511):319–23.
8. Shoemaker WC. Editorial: multiple injuries and multiple organ failure. Crit Care Med. 1973;1(3):157.
9. Trubuhovich RV. Acute brain swelling. Int Anesthesiol Clin. 1979;17(2–3):77–31.
10. Safar P, Bleyaert A, Nemoto EM, Moossy J, Snyder JV. Resuscitation after global brain ischemia-anoxia. Crit Care Med. 1978;6(4):215–27.

11. Laurence DR, Berman E, Scragg JN, Adams EB. A clinical trial of chlorpromazine against barbiturates in tetanus. Lancet. 1958;1(7028):987–91.
12. Hill GL. Surgeon scientist: adventures in surgical research. Auckland: Random House; 2006.
13. Beddoe AH, Streat SJ, Hill GL. Evaluation of an in-vivo prompt gamma neutron activation facility for body composition studies in critically ill intensive care patients: results on 41 normals. Metabolism. 1984;33:270–80.
14. Streat SJ, Beddoe AH, Hill GL. Measurement of total body water in intensive care patients with fluid overload. Metabolism. 1985;34:688–94.
15. Streat SJ, Beddoe AH, Hill GL. Aggressive nutritional support does not prevent protein loss despite fat gain in septic intensive care patients. J Trauma. 1987;27(3):262–6.
16. Clark MA, Plank LD, Connolly AB, Streat SJ, Hill AA, Gupta R, Monk DN, Shenkin A, Hill GL. Effect of a chimeric antibody to tumor necrosis factor-α on cytokine and physiologic responses in patients with severe sepsis – a randomized clinical trial. Crit Care Med. 1998;26(10):1650–9.
17. Cassell J, Buchman TG, Streat S, Stewart RM. Surgeons, Intensivists and the covenant of care – administrative models and values affecting care at the end of life – Updated. Crit Care Med. 2003;31(5):1551–9.
18. Cuthbertson SJ, Margetts MA, Streat SJ. Bereavement follow-up after critical illness. Crit Care Med. 2000;28(4):1196–201.
19. Breen J. Road safety advocacy. BMJ. 2004;328(7444):888–90.
20. Key R, Cuthbertson S, Streat S. How everybody benefits from follow-up after critical illness. Aust Crit Care. 1997;10(1):27.
21. Trubuhovich RV, Judson JA. Intensive care in New Zealand. Auckland: Cox & Dawes; 2001.
22. Young P, Saxena M, Bellomo R, Freebairn R, Hammond N, van Haren F, Holliday M, Henderson S, Mackle D, McArthur C, McGuinness S, Myburgh J, Weatherall M, Webb S, Beasley R, HEAT Investigators and the Australian and New Zealand Intensive Care Society Clinical Trials Group. Acetaminophen for fever in critically Ill patients with suspected infection. N Engl J Med. 2015;373(23):2215–24.
23. Nichol A, French C, Little L, Haddad S, Presneill J, Arabi Y, Bailey M, Cooper DJ, Duranteau J, Huet O, Mak A, McArthur C, Pettilä V, Skrifvars M, Vallance S, Varma D, Wills J, Bellomo R; EPO-TBI Investigators and the ANZICS Clinical Trials Group. Erythropoietin in traumatic brain injury (EPO-TBI): a double-blind randomised controlled trial. Lancet. 2015. pii: S0140-6736(15)00386-4.
24. Young P, Bailey M, Beasley R, Henderson S, Mackle D, McArthur C, McGuinness S, Mehrtens J, Myburgh J, Psirides A, Reddy S, Bellomo R, SPLIT Investigators, ANZICS CTG. Effect of a buffered crystalloid solution vs saline on acute kidney injury among patients in the intensive care unit: the SPLIT randomized clinical trial. JAMA. 2015;314(16):1701–10.
25. ARISE Investigators, ANZICS Clinical Trials Group, Peake SL, Delaney A, Bailey M, Bellomo R, Cameron PA, Cooper DJ, Higgins AM, Holdgate A, Howe BD, Webb SA, Williams P. Goal-directed resuscitation for patients with early septic shock. N Engl J Med. 2014;371(16):1496–506.
26. Holcomb BW, Wheeler AP, Ely EW. New ways to reduce unnecessary variation and improve outcomes in the intensive care unit. Curr Opin Crit Care. 2001;7:304–11.
27. Kern H, Kox WJ. Impact of standard procedures and clinical standards on cost-effectiveness and intensive care unit performance in adult patients after cardiac surgery. Intensive Care Med. 1999;25:1367–73.
28. Morris AH. Developing and implementing computerized protocols for standardization of clinical decisions. Ann Intern Med. 2000;132:373–83.
29. Gane E, McCall J, Streat S, Gunn K, Yeong ML, Fitt S, Keenan D, Munn S. Liver Transplantation in New Zealand. The first 4 years. N Z Med J. 2002;115(1159):U120.
30. Plank LD, Metzger DJ, McCall JL, Barclay KL, Gane EJ, Streat SJ, Munn SR, Hill GL. Sequential changes in the metabolic response to orthotopic liver transplantation during the first year after operation. Ann Surg. 2001;234(2):245–55.

31. Munn SR, Evans HM, Gane EJ. The New Zealand liver transplant unit: Auckland District Health Board. Clin Transpl. 2014:91–8.
32. Streat S, Munn S. Health economics and health technology assessment: perspectives from Australia and New Zealand. Crit Care Clin. 2012;28(1):125–33.
33. Taylor C, Graham J, Potts HW, Richards MA, Ramirez AJ. Changes in mental health of UK hospital consultants since the mid-1990s. Lancet. 2005;366:742–4.
34. Australian and New Zealand Intensive Care Society. The ANZICS statement on death and organ donation (Edition 3.2). Melbourne: ANZICS, 2013. Available via www.anzics.com.au. Accessed 11th Dec 2015.
35. Australian and New Zealand Intensive Care Society. ANZICS statement on care and decision-making at the end of life for the critically Ill (Edition 1.0). Melbourne, ANZICS, 2014. Available via www.anzics.com.au. Accessed 11th Dec 2015.

Chapter 15
Future of Critical Care Medicine

W. Andrew Kofke and Guy Kositratna

It started in 1967, a buddy Mike Ruscher says to the 15-year-old me (WAK) that there's a new volunteer ambulance service starting in Adamsburg; let's join. The notion of a couple of teens being able to run in an EMS system, with only Red Cross first aid training, indicates the progress that has been made since then. My experience started in a converted hearse, progressing to the rudiments of EMS as we became among the first EMTs certified in Pennsylvania (Fig. 15.1). As things progressed, advanced cardiac techniques, for that day, were being brought on scene as CCU nurses joined us. Along the way, advances in trauma management and BLS were growing. Jaws of Life was introduced. Then came medical school, 1974–1978. Handheld calculators were hot. On to residency in anesthesiology at MGH, 36-h days were commonplace. Notably there were no pulse oximeters, blood pressure was measured manually every 5 min, and only the occasional anesthesia machine had an oxygen analyzer. The resident's monitoring via esophageal stethoscope was the patient's lifeline. The single available fiber-optic bronchoscope was only allowed to be used by ICU fellows, and patients were being mechanically ventilated on the floor with no alarms. Found dead in bed was not uncommon. Patient safety practices were not here yet. I knew of a patient undergoing cholecystectomy who had already had the thing removed at another hospital (buried in the records) but, due to fear of the surgical hierarchy, dared not speak; after all these were Ivy League surgeons! (Fig. 15.2).

Things have progressed quite a bit over the past 35 years, and this cumulative experience perhaps can allow some forecasting as to the future of critical care. However, caution is needed as the slope of progress may not be linear – if exponential, then it may ascend at a dizzying pace.

W.A. Kofke, MD, MBA, FCCM, FNCS (✉) • G. Kositratna, MD
Department of Anesthesiology and Critical Care, University of Pennsylvania,
7 Dulles Building 3400 Spruce Street, Philadelphia, PA 19104-4283, USA
e-mail: william.kofke@uphs.upenn.edu

© Springer International Publishing Switzerland 2016
D. Crippen (ed.), *The Intensivist's Challenge: Aging and Career Growth in a High-Stress Medical Specialty*, DOI 10.1007/978-3-319-30454-0_15

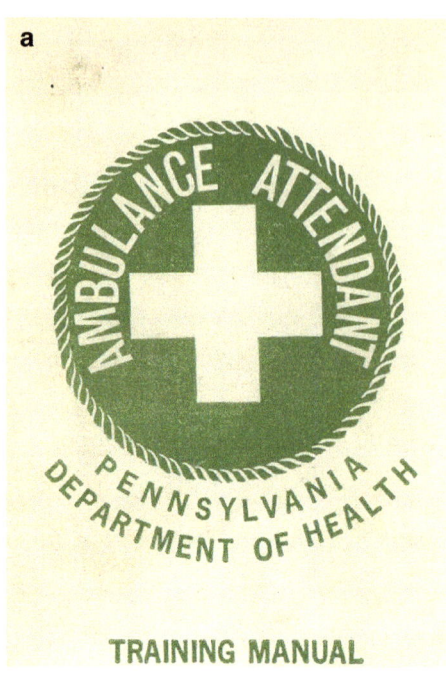

RESUSCITATION & CARE OF THE UNCONSCIOUS PATIENT

Prepared by

Peter Safar, M.D., and Richard Brose, F.A.P.H.A.
Department of Anesthesiology
U. of Pittsburgh School of Medicine

General Remarks

Every year in the United States approximately 90,000 people die from accidents and 500,000 die from heart attacks. Among the deaths occurring outside of hospitals, a number would have been reversible by modern resuscitation techniques. For instance, many of the 40,000 patients who die annually from highway accidents do not die because of their primary injury (e. g., head injury, crushing injury of the chest), but because of airway obstruction, respiratory depression or shock. These patients, particularly the unconscious ones, often need correction of the airway obstruction and artificial ventilation at the scene of the accident and continued resuscitative efforts during transportation to the hospital.

Many unconscious patients do not require artificial ventilation, but merely proper positioning to allow adequate natural breathing through an open air passage. A good example is the patient with a head injury, his fate often lying in your hands. His brain may suffer irreparable damage within a few minutes if you do not provide for constant adequate breathing.

The well-informed ambulance attendant confronted with an unconscious patient should first make an effort to establish breathing and circulation at the scene of the accident, instead of rushing the dying or dead victim as rapidly as possible to the hospital without resuscitative efforts.

TRAINING MANUAL

Fig. 15.1 (**a**) Cover of EMT textbook used for an innovative course to train emergency medical technicians in Pennsylvania in the late 1960s. (**b**) First page of Chap. 2 in EMT textbook dealing with the unconscious patient and first authored by Peter Safar, one of the major leaders in early EMS, intensive care, and cardiopulmonary resuscitation

In this chapter, we review many of these new research areas and speculate as to how they may eventually translate to clinical care. The topic is broad so the review is necessarily incomplete. The primary focus will be on neuro-ICU but with some discussion of general critical care.

Genomics

Genomic variation [1] and interfering RNA [2] technology foretell a day when the human genome will become a routine part of history and physical examination. Since identification of the entire genomes of many humans has been accomplished [3], the future of critical care medicine will likely see patients arriving to the hospital with their entire genomes on record. The individual genomic pattern would allow clinicians to anticipate the course of disease, accurately prognosticate outcome, tailor the treatment that most fits each particular patient, and even foretell susceptibility to complications [4]. Such futuristic concepts underlie the work in the

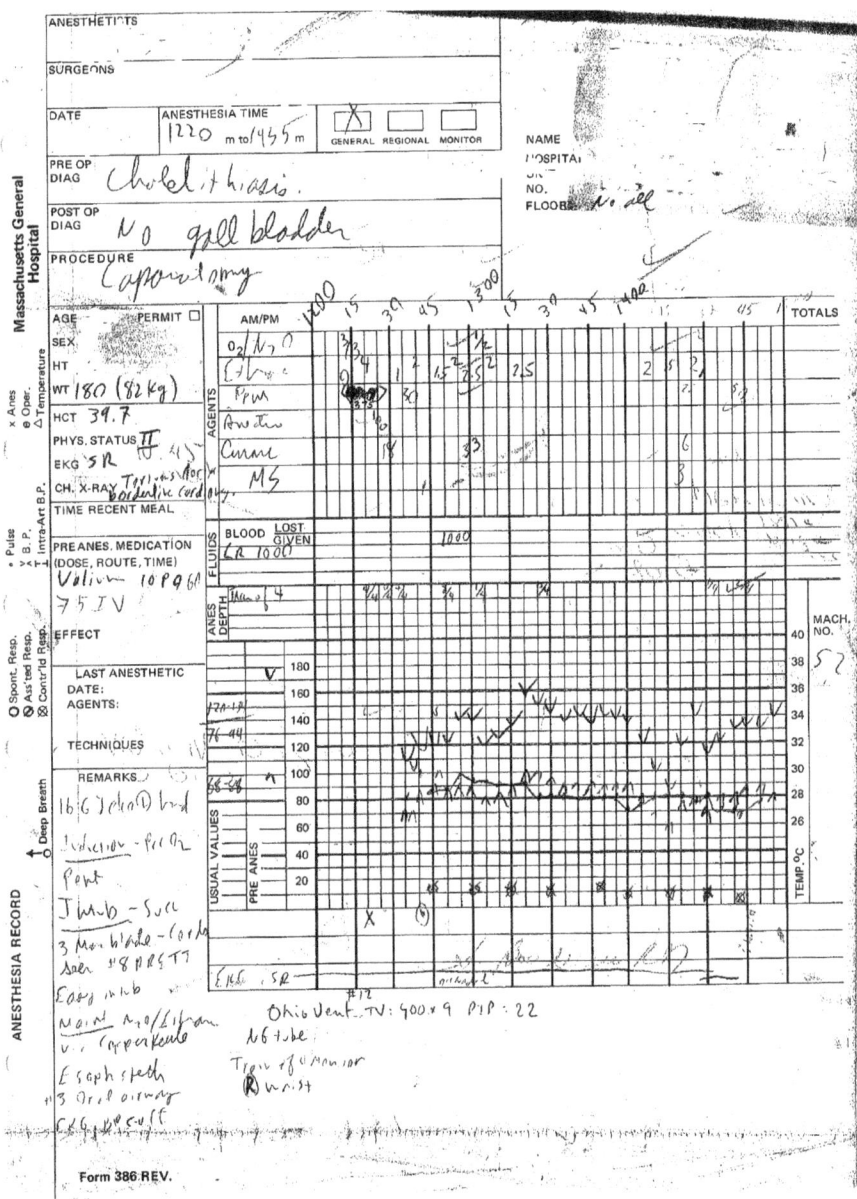

Fig. 15.2 Anesthesia record provides an example of anesthesia and critical care technology and safety culture before 1980. Note lack of pulse oximetry, end-tidal gas monitoring, inspiratory oxygen assessment, and also the use of esophageal stethoscope as a primary monitor of ventilation, heart tones, and contractility. Finally this record depicts the results of a culture of career-fear on patient safety

EMERGE network [5] with many early examples of this. Furthermore, this information will certainly bring us a possibility to modify individual's genotype, genomic regulation, or phenotype based on what is seen during the course of treatment or based on specific responses to interventions. A series of annual reviews have underscored these issues [6–8].

Genomic information will likely relate to sedative and analgesic tolerance [9–13], pain tolerance [14] and anticipated needs for postoperative pain control regimens, and possibly susceptibility to addiction [15–26]. Moreover, SNPs are now being described in humans regarding genetic predisposition to postoperative nausea and vomiting [27, 28], malignant hyperthermia [29], and cognitive dysfunction [30].

Genetic influences on pharmacokinetics have become reasonably well known for a handful of antihypertensive drugs as they relate to genetic effects on metabolism (e.g., hydralazine) [31] and perioperative drugs [32–34]. Certainly, genetic factors are known for such entities as pseudocholinesterase deficiency [35], the interaction of thiopental with porphyria [36], or the genetics of malignant hyperthermia [29, 37]. Cytochrome P450 is important in the metabolism of many drugs including anesthetics. These genomic variations have been reported to impact on the metabolism of midazolam [38] and opioids [32, 33]. Clinical relevance is made manifest in a report of genomic differences with cytochrome contributing to mortality from nonmedical fentanyl ingestion [39]. Multiple other effects of genetic variation on anesthetic metabolism and side effects have been reviewed [40]. It is clear that increased information will become available with respect to SNPs, arrays of SNPs, and other causes of genetic variation and their impact on sedative and other drug metabolism [37].

One group reports that up to 10 % or more of genes undergo alteration in expression after brain ischemia [41, 42]. In humans, alteration in expression of genes responsible for the inflammatory response has similarly been reported after stroke [43, 44]. Many others report increased risk of stroke associated with different genotypes. Thus, the effect of one's genomic inheritance on predisposition to stroke and susceptibility to its sequelae may be an important piece of information that will guide future therapies [45–58].

Gene association studies with stroke are just one example of the role of genomics in defining a given medical risk. Such studies are burgeoning regarding a host of medical conditions. There have been some studies showing statistical associations between specific SNPs and postoperative complications [59]. Specific examples include renal failure [60, 61], posttransplant kidney infection [62], total hip arthroplasty failure [63, 64], allograft dysfunction [65], pain intensity and analgesic requirements [66–72], vasopressor requirements [73], myocardial infarction [74], inflammatory response [75], thromboembolism [76, 77], stroke [78], and vascular graft patency [79, 80]. These studies will undoubtedly contribute to risk assessment in individual patients and lead to new therapeutic strategies designed to minimize perioperative complications.

Omic Signatures

Characterization of the entire genomes of many humans has been accomplished [3]. This, combined with the above noted material, indicates a future, which will encompass patients arriving for surgery with their entire genomes on record. This will likely also include other personal "omics" profiling. Applied across a population, including critical care patients, this suggests characterization of the genome, epigenome, transcriptome, proteome, cytokine-ome, metabolome, autoantibody-ome, and microbiome (gut, urine, nose, tongue, skin) for possibly billions of individuals. With this we will have a large amount of impressively big data (e.g., a million genes and other -omic information in millions to billions of people). One hoped for consequence of this will be an ability to predict and monitor diseases resulting in personalized therapies identified from big data analyses.

The gut microbiome has been described as a *forgotten organ* [81] and has also been hypothesized to control the mammalian immune system [82]. Cumulative evidence suggests its importance beyond this whereby the microbiome certainly plays a pivotal role in maintaining homeostasis of the entire body. Therefore, quantitative and functional alterations of such microorganisms will exert a great impact on human health in many ways. Preclinical studies indicate an important role of the microbiome in resistance to infection and proper cytokine response [83, 84]. Conversely, microbes can alter their own virulence by sensing the host environment and other bacteria in the vicinity, resulting in a transformation into a more pathognomonic phenotype. The new pathologic bacteria then cause sepsis and remote organ dysfunction even without systemic dissemination of the pathogen itself [85–87]. Furthermore, probiotics can improve intestinal environment. Probiotics reduce mortality rate, decrease bacteremia, and ameliorate gut epithelial homeostasis following experimental sepsis [88]. They can also attenuate growth of intestinal bacteria which consecutively limits endotoxin production and reduces the risk of bacteremia [89]. Further studies targeting the gut are still required and this will be a prime research interest in the near future.

Stem Cells

Over the last two decades, research in regenerative medicine has emphasized cell-based therapy as a probable therapeutic alternative for many diseases. Preclinical studies in traumatic brain injury models have demonstrated the migration and proliferation of progenitor cells into the damaged brain areas, resulting in protective effects via cell replacement, gene and protein transfer, and modulation of anti-inflammatory and growth factors [90]. Mesenchymal stem cells (MSCs) are another promising therapeutic option as they can be successfully isolated and cultured. A recent human study has shown positive results of the MSC transplant for its safety and efficacy among patients with ischemic stroke [91]. Also, injecting the MSCs into the intervertebral disc of those suffering form discogenic back pain may improve pain and function up to 2 years post-procedure [92]. Other non-neurologic applications of stem cells are likely to emerge.

Indeed, one further implication is that critical care physicians will encounter more patients having a stem cell transplant or encounter those who have had it earlier in life. The care of such patients will be more intricate as the physiologic milieu of the implantation will definitely become a primary concern.

Sepsis

To date, many phase III clinical trials have failed to target the host septic inflammatory response such as anti-TNF or APC [93–95], whereas, simply controlling the source of infection is still mandatory. It is believed that pathogen toxins are cleared mainly by hepatic uptake and biliary excretion [96] in which the LDL receptor (LDLR) may play an important role as most of the toxins contain lipid components [97]. Mechanisms by which the body eliminates the toxins including the role of PCSK9 might be new strategies for future sepsis treatment [98]. In addition, development of new therapeutic strategies aimed at modulating the innate immunity (activations of complements, phagocytes, and natural killer cells) is conceivable and many of which are under investigations [99–101]. Another aspect that will be scrutinized further is the management of vascular leakage which may be impacted by vasopressor choice [102–107] or endothelial factors (sphingosine-1-phosphate) [108–113] that may be therapeutic targets.

ARDS

Multiple studies are ongoing, further evaluating and refining tidal volumes, airway pressures [113–121], management of ventilator dyssynchrony, optimal use of neuromuscular blockade, and prone positioning [122–127].

CT scan is presently the gold standard for assessing the effect of recruitment [128, 129] but with transport issues. Electrical impedance tomography (EIT) may be more advantageous as it is a real-time monitoring device proven comparable to the CT for the assessment of changes in gas volume and gas distribution within the lungs [130–136]. The EIT may provide some benefits as it is noninvasive and can be used continuously at bedside.

Neuroprotection

Notwithstanding ample promising preclinical work, there are very few neuroprotectant strategies that have sustained scrutiny in clinical trials. Techniques which have been studied and may have a role in future neuroprotection schemes include hypothermia [137–143] and hibernation [144–147]. These notions form the basis for ongoing research to develop suspended animation methods, with overt intent to copy hibernation biochemistry and physiology [145, 146, 148, 149] translated to attenuate problems in human neuroprotection.

Several reports suggest that infrared light can be used to penetrate the skull to improve tissue energetics, notwithstanding an anaerobic condition. Shining low-level infrared light at a specific wavelength improves ATP production in neuronal culture [150] and improves neurological outcome in animal stroke models [151–153] with some promise in clinical studies [154].

Multimodality Approach to Neuroprotection

Establishing efficacy of new neuroprotective therapies in neurocritical care and stroke has proven to be an exercise in futility [155]. Over 2000 completed clinical trials are listed on the Internet Stroke Trials Registry [156] with few apparent reproducible results of any demonstrable efficacy in the acute context. However, these many negative studies belie the supportive basic laboratory studies that justified the time and enormous expense for such attempted translational clinical trials. We provide a rationale to suggest that such results, in retrospect, are altogether predictable and suggest an explanatory model for such reproducible futility in a complex biological system. Many of the points discussed are supported in an editorial by Grotta [155]. It is to be expected that these issues will eventually lead to a commonplace approach to use multimodal therapies for neuroprotection. Donnan [157] in the 2007 Feinberg lecture suggests: "We have reached a stage at which research in this area should stop altogether or radical new approaches adopted." The new approaches may include a reevaluation of prospective randomized studies as the only path to new knowledge. A rationale for this approach and suggested methodology is advocated by Kofke [158].

Spinal Cord Injury Neuroprotection

Current research suggests several approaches likely to be translated eventually to clinical care. These include pharmacological therapies [159], surgical decompression [159, 160], and hypothermia [161–163].

Mesquita et al. are presently developing a near-infrared spectroscopy-based device which could be placed in a manner similar to an epidural catheter to yield continuous real-time spinal cord blood flow information. This could have a dramatic impact on the management of patients presenting with spinal cord injury or spinal cord ischemia [164].

Stem Cell Therapy This is based on the use of embryonic stem cells or progenitor cells from other sources such as the bone marrow to promote regeneration of cells and remyelination [165–168]. Animal studies support the feasibility of this approach, showing the capability of embryonic stem cells to develop into glial cells and into neural cells which make synaptic contacts [165]. In addition to these sources, the nervous system itself may also be a source of endogenous stem cells [165].

Genomic Therapy Preclinical studies suggest a role for siRNAs in potentiating repair after SCI [169]. After spinal cord injury, astrocyte activation promotes glial scar formation.

Neurotrophin Therapy [159] A variety of approaches are currently being explored including cytokine blockade [170], implantation of trophin-producing cells [168, 171], viral gene transfer [172], and implantation of stem cell progenitors of glial cells [173].

Overall, spinal cord injury, once considered a hopeless injury, now has ongoing research which suggests, likely administered as a multimodality battery, that there may be effective therapies eventually available.

Technology

Monitoring

Neuromonitoring has long been an area of active research and clinical contributions in critical care.

Continuous regional blood flow and metabolic rate monitoring, long a holy grail of neuromonitoring, should eventually be realized as a clinical reality. Currently attractive noninvasive methods tend to be based on near-infrared spectroscopy (NIRS) with other invasive techniques that may also be useful. Researchers are reporting use of NIRS to facilitate continuous bedside rCBF monitoring. NIRS-based diffuse correlation spectroscopy (*DCS*) and diffuse reflectance spectroscopy (*DRS*) and NIRS-based ICG blood flow index (*BFI*) and absolute CBF hold significant promise as bedside monitors of rCBF and metabolic rate (*CMRO2*). DCS combined with ICG offers the potential for a truly continuous rCBF, OEF, and CMRO2 monitor [174–182]. Acousto-optic techniques are also available which can be used to measure relative changes in CBF. Validation studies are ongoing [183, 184].

Robots: Feedback Loop Controllers

BIS and patient state index (PSI) monitors have undergone extensive evaluation as monitors of depth of hypnosis with reasonable evidence for a role in some neurosurgical settings [185]. Recent early work [186] in this area suggests that added depth of analgesia monitoring will also eventually be developed and validated. Studies have been done on facial EMG, palmar conductance [187, 188], and pupillometry [189] with reasonable results, suggesting that such monitoring should be clinically feasible for future applications. The Analgoscore is another means of monitoring intraoperative pain by the application of an algorithm to blood pressure and heart rate data [190]. The availability of depth of hypnosis, analgesia, and neuromuscular blockade, along with cardiovascular monitoring, will then enable the intensivists to precisely titrate the anesthetic drug as a "magic bullet" directed to that element of the anesthetic state most in need of attention [191, 192]. Researchers at McGill University have described such a system which they have named McSleepy [191, 192]. This group is also exploring the performance of a robotic intubation system called the Kepler intubation system [193, 194].

Multimodality Brain Monitoring

Brain tissue pO2 (pbO2), microdialysis, and blood flow methods are receiving significant attention presently. There is ample retrospective evidence to associate a low pbO2, low CBF [191, 192, 195–197], and elevated lactate pyruvate ratio with poor outcome [198–201], and certainly it makes physiologic sense. It seems reasonable to expect that these monitors will eventually find a place in titration of the physiologic contributors' secondary processes in brain injury. Multimodality monitoring has recently been evaluated in a consensus statement [202].

Exhaled Gas Monitoring

Previously the province of nonportable GC mass spectrometry types of equipment, improved sensor, and computing technology has resulted in capability to place a highly sensitive array of chemical sensors in exhalation tubing of a patient to make significant physiologic inferences [203]. Currently published examples suggest an ability to detect bacterial pneumonia [204], sinusitis [205], asthma [206], aerodigestive tract tumor cells [207], lung cancer [208], and tuberculosis [209]. The technology has been reported to be able to detect lipid peroxidation in food [210]. Given that lipid peroxidation [211–214] or perhaps release of other volatile organic compounds occurs with ischemia, it becomes plausible to suggest that this technology will have a place in screening for immediate evidence of ongoing cerebral (or other organ) ischemia in neuroanesthesia and neurocritical care.

Telemedicine

Remote ICU methods are receiving increasing attention. They can either involve a robot with a screenshot of a remote physician [215] or have multiply wired rooms with monitoring and remote availability of ICU physicians and nurses [216, 217]. This technology is just beginning but can be expected to have an increased value in the ICU of the future.

Pharmacology

Fast on Fast off

Work has been ongoing for decades in an effort to elucidate mechanisms of anesthesia. Implicit in such work has been the assumption that induction of anesthesia and emergence are equal and opposite biological processes. However, Kelz et al. suggest that the neural substrates that underlie induction and emergence are different and present the concept of neural inertia in transitions in levels of consciousness [218, 219]. In their work, they describe the role of the endogenous orexin system in impacting emergence from, but not entry into, the anesthetized state [220]. This then suggests that future pharmacologic work in this area may lead to methods to manipulate the process of emergence from anesthesia such that, rather than awaiting dissipation or antagonizing the induction anesthetic drugs, specific manipulation of the neural substrates of emergence from anesthesia will lead to faster more reliable emergence from anesthesia after neurosurgical procedures.

Another potential advance is the advent of very short-acting anesthetic agents. This is best illustrated with remifentanil for analgesia. Work is underway, suggesting a future similarly short-acting context-insensitive benzodiazepine hypnotic, remimazolam [221, 222]. Development of a comparably short-acting neuromuscular blocking drug would then have the stage set for titratable context-insensitive sedation paradigms in the ICU.

Summary

This chapter has reviewed some current research in areas relevant to critical care and neurocritical care. Some clinical problem areas have been suggested as important objects of research with a distillation of nascent work, which can be reasonably anticipated to translate to clinical care. If these speculations are borne out, the ICU of the future will indeed look a good deal different and better than the one of today.

References

1. Reynolds A, Leake D, Boese Q, Scaringe S, Marshall WS, Khvorova A, et al. Rational siRNA design for RNA interference. Nat Biotechnol. 2004;22(3):326–30.
2. NIGMS. The New Genetics Bethesda: NIGMS. 2007 [updated 27 June 2007; cited 2008 6 May 2008]. Available from: http://publications.nigms.nih.gov/thenewgenetics/glossary.html.
3. Chi KR. The year of sequencing. Nat Methods. 2008;5(1):11–4.
4. Allen PD. Anesthesia and the human genome project: the quest for accurate prediction of drug responses. Anesthesiology. 2005;102(3):494–5.

5. McCarty C, Chisholm R, Chute C, Kullo I, Jarvik G, Larson E, et al. The eMERGE network: a consortium of biorepositories linked to electronic medical records data for conducting genomic studies. BMC Med Genomics. 2011;4(1):13.
6. Hegele RA, Dichgans M, Hegele RA, Dichgans M. Update on the genetics of stroke and cerebrovascular disease 2007. Stroke. 2008;39(2):252–4.
7. Dichgans M, Hegele RA, Dichgans M, Hegele RA. Update on the genetics of stroke and cerebrovascular disease 2006. Stroke. 2007;38(2):216–8.
8. Alberts MJ, Tournier-Lasserve E, Alberts MJ, Tournier-Lasserve E. Update on the genetics of stroke and cerebrovascular disease 2004. Stroke. 2005;36(2):179–81.
9. Liem EB, Lin CM, Suleman MI, Doufas AG, Gregg RG, Veauthier JM, et al. Anesthetic requirement is increased in redheads. Anesthesiology. 2004;101(2):279–83.
10. Rajaram S, Sedensky MM, Morgan PG. Unc-1: a stomatin homologue controls sensitivity to volatile anesthetics in Caenorhabditis elegans. Proc Natl Acad Sci U S A. 1998;95(15): 8761–6.
11. Kayser EB, Morgan PG, Sedensky MM. GAS-1: a mitochondrial protein controls sensitivity to volatile anesthetics in the nematode Caenorhabditis elegans. Anesthesiology. 1999;90(2):545–54.
12. Sato Y, Seo N, Kobayashi E. Genetic background differences between FVB and C57BL/6 mice affect hypnotic susceptibility to pentobarbital, ketamine and nitrous oxide, but not isoflurane. Acta Anaesthesiol Scand. 2006;50(5):553–6.
13. Mulholland CV, Somogyi AA, Barratt DT, Coller JK, Hutchinson MR, Jacobson GM, et al. Association of innate immune single-nucleotide polymorphisms with the electroencephalogram during desflurane general anaesthesia. J Mol Neurosci. 2014;52(4):497–506.
14. Liem EB, Joiner TV, Tsueda K, Sessler DI. Increased sensitivity to thermal pain and reduced subcutaneous lidocaine efficacy in redheads. Anesthesiology. 2005;102(3):509–14.
15. Boules ML, Botros SKA, Shaheen IA, Hamed MA. Association of u-opioid receptor gene polymorphism (A118G) with variations in fentanyl analgesia consumption after total abdominal hysterectomy in female Egyptian patients. Comp Clin Pathol. 2014;1–6.
16. Kambur O, Kaunisto MA, Tikkanen E, Leal SM, Ripatti S, Kalso EA. Effect of catechol-o-methyltransferase-gene (COMT) variants on experimental and acute postoperative pain in 1,000 women undergoing surgery for breast cancer. Anesthesiology. 2013;119(6):1422–33.
17. Sia AT, Lim Y, Lim ECP, Ocampo CE, Lim WY, Cheong P, et al. Influence of mu-opioid receptor variant on morphine use and self-rated pain following abdominal hysterectomy. J Pain. 2013;14(10):1045–52.
18. Liao Q, Chen DJ, Zhang F, Li L, Hu R, Tang YZ, et al. Effect of CYP3A4*18B polymorphisms and interactions with OPRM1 A118G on postoperative fentanyl requirements in patients undergoing radical gastrectomy. Mol Med Rep. 2013;7(3):901–8.
19. Duan G, Xiang G, Zhang X, Yuan R, Zhan H, Qi D. A single-nucleotide polymorphism in SCN9A may decrease postoperative pain sensitivity in the general population. Anesthesiology. 2013;118(2):436–42.
20. Storm H, Stå̩en R, Klepstad P, Skorpen F, Qvigstad E, Rå†der J. Nociceptive stimuli responses at different levels of general anaesthesia and genetic variability. Acta Anaesthesiol Scand. 2013;57(1):89–99.
21. Ochroch EA, Vachani A, Gottschalk A, Kanetsky PA. Natural variation in the mu-opioid gene OPRM1 predicts increased pain on third day after thoracotomy. Clin J Pain. 2012;28(9):747–54.
22. Camorcia M, Capogna G, Stirparo S, Berritta C, Blouin JL, Landau R. Effect of u-opioid receptor A118G polymorphism on the ED50 of epidural sufentanil for labor analgesia. Int J Obstet Anesth. 2012;21(1):40–4.
23. Zhang W, Yuan JJ, Kan QC, Zhang LR, Chang YZ, Wang ZY, et al. Influence of CYP3A5*3 polymorphism and interaction between CYP3A5*3 and CYP3A4*1G polymorphisms on post-operative fentanyl analgesia in Chinese patients undergoing gynaecological surgery. Eur J Anaesthesiol. 2011;28(4):245–50.

24. Hackel D, Krug SM, Sauer RS, Mousa SA, Bocker A, Pflucke D, et al. Transient opening of the perineurial barrier for analgesic drug delivery. Proc Natl Acad Sci U S A. 2012;109(29):E2018–27.

25. Yang CH, Huang HW, Chen KH, Chen YS, Sheen-Chen SM, Lin CR. Antinociceptive potentiation and attenuation of tolerance by intrathecal Î²-arrestin 2 small interfering RNA in rats. Br J Anaesth. 2011;107(5):774–81.

26. Dray A. Neuropathic pain: emerging treatments. Br J Anaesth. 2008;101(1):48–58.

27. Sugino S, Hayase T, Higuchi M, Saito K, Moriya H, Kumeta Y, et al. Association of u-opioid receptor gene (OPRM1) haplotypes with postoperative nausea and vomiting. Exp Brain Res. 2014.

28. Ma XX, Chen QX, Wu SJ, Hu Y, Fang XM. Polymorphisms of the HTR3B gene are associated with post-surgery emesis in a Chinese Han population. J Clin Pharm Ther. 2013;38(2):150–5.

29. Brandom BW, Bina S, Wong CA, Wallace T, Visoiu M, Isackson PJ, et al. Ryanodine receptor type 1 gene variants in the malignant hyperthermia-susceptible population of the United States. Anesth Analg. 2013;116(5):1078–86.

30. Cai Y, Hu H, Liu P, Feng G, Dong W, Yu B, et al. Association between the apolipoprotein E4 and postoperative cognitive dysfunction in elderly patients undergoing intravenous anesthesia and inhalation anesthesia. Anesthesiology. 2012;116(1):84–93.

31. Ludden TM, McNay Jr JL, Shepherd AM, Lin MS, Ludden TM, McNay Jr JL, et al. Variability of plasma hydralazine concentrations in male hypertensive patients. Arthritis Rheum. 1981;24(8):987–93.

32. Lambert DG. Pharmacogenomics. Anaesthesia Intensive Care Med. 2013;14(4):166–8.

33. Cohen M, Sadhasivam S, Vinks AA. Pharmacogenetics in perioperative medicine. Curr Opin Anaesthesiol. 2012;25(4):419–27.

34. Fernandez Robles CR, Degnan M, Candiotti KA. Pain and genetics. Curr Opin Anaesthesiol. 2012;25(4):444–9.

35. Hanel HK, Viby-Mogensen J, de Muckadell OB, Hanel HK, Viby-Mogensen J, de Muckadell OB. Serum cholinesterase variants in the Danish population. Acta Anaesthesiol Scand. 1978;22(5):505–7.

36. Dundee JW, Mc CW, Mc LG, Dundee JW, McCleery WN, McLoughlin G. The hazard of thiopental anaesthesia in porphyria. Anesth Analg. 1962;41:567–74.

37. Galley HF, Mahdy A, Lowes DA. Pharmacogenetics and anesthesiologists. Pharmacogenomics. 2005;6(8):849–56.

38. He P, Court MH, Greenblatt DJ, von Moltke LL. Factors influencing midazolam hydroxylation activity in human liver microsomes. Drug Metab Dispos. 2006;34(7):1198–207.

39. Jin M, Gock SB, Jannetto PJ, Jentzen JM, Wong SH. Pharmacogenomics as molecular autopsy for forensic toxicology: genotyping cytochrome P450 3A4*1B and 3A5*3 for 25 fentanyl cases. J Anal Toxicol. 2005;29(7):590–8.

40. Palmer SN, Giesecke NM, Body SC, Shernan SK, Fox AA, Collard CD. Pharmacogenetics of anesthetic and analgesic agents. Anesthesiology. 2005;102(3):663–71.

41. Tang Y, Lu A, Aronow B, Wagner K, Sharp F. Genomic responses of the brain to ischemic stroke, intracerebral hemorrhage, kainate seizures, hypoglycemia, and hypoxia. Eur J Neurosci. 2002;15(12):1937–52.

42. Schwarz D, Barry G, Mackay K, Manu F, Naeve G, Vana A, et al. Identification of differentially expressed genes induced by transient ischemic stroke. Mol Brain Res. 2002;101(1–2):12–22.

43. Tang Y, Xu H, Du X, Lit L, Walker W, Lu A, et al. Gene expression in blood changes rapidly in neutrophils and monocytes after ischemic stroke in humans: a microarray study. J Cereb Blood Flow Metab. 2006;26(8):1089–102.

44. Sharp FR, Xu H, Lit L, Walker W, Pinter J, Apperson M, et al. Genomic profiles of stroke in blood. Stroke. 2007;38(2 Suppl):691–3.

45. Kitagawa K, Matsumoto M, Kuwabara K, Ohtsuki T, Hori M. Delayed, but marked, expression of apolipoprotein E is involved in tissue clearance after cerebral infarction. J Cereb Blood Flow Metab. 2001;21(10):1199–207.

46. Panahian N, Yoshiura M, Maines M. Overexpression of heme oxygenase-1 is neuroprotective in a model of permanent middle cerebral artery occlusion in transgenic mice. J Neurochem. 1999;72(3):1187–203.
47. Lukkarinen J, Kauppinen R, Grohn O, Oja J, Sinervirta R, Jarvinen A, et al. Neuroprotective role of ornithine decarboxylase activation in transient focal cerebral ischaemia: a study using ornithine decarboxylase-overexpressing transgenic rats. Eur J Neurosci. 1998;10(6):2046–55.
48. Weisbrot-Lefkowitz M, Reuhl K, Perry B, Chan P, Inouye M, Mirochnitchenko O. Overexpression of human glutathione peroxidase protects transgenic mice against focal cerebral ischemia/reperfusion damage. Mol Brain Res. 1998;53(1–2):333–8.
49. Rajdev S, Hara K, Kokubo Y, Mestril R, Dillmann W, Weinstein P, et al. Mice overexpressing rat heat shock protein 70 are protected against cerebral infarction. Ann Neurol. 2000;47(6):782–91.
50. Sharp F, Bergeron M, Bernaudin M. Hypoxia-inducible factor in brain. Adv Exp Med Biol. 2001;502:273–91.
51. Siren A, Ehrenreich H. Erythropoietin--a novel concept for neuroprotection. Eur Arch Psychiatry Clin Neurosci. 2001;251(4):179–84.
52. Schaller B, Bahr M, Buchfelder M. Pathophysiology of brain ischemia: penumbra, gene expression, and future therapeutic options. Eur Neurol. 2005;54(4):179–80.
53. Kofke W, Konitzer P, Meng Q, Guo J, Cheung A. Effect of apolipoprotein E genotype on NSE and S-100 levels after cardiac and vascular surgery. Anesth Analg. 2004;99:1323–5.
54. Yenari M, Dumas T, Sapolsky R, Steinberg G. Gene therapy for treatment of cerebral ischemia using defective herpes simplex viral vectors. Neurol Res. 2001;23(5):543–52.
55. Gidday J, Fitzgibbons J, Shah A, Park T. Neuroprotection from ischemic brain injury by hypoxic preconditioning in the neonatal rat. Neurosci Lett. 1994;168(1–2):221–4.
56. Koistinaho J, Hökfelt T. Altered gene expression in brain ischemia. Neuroreport. 1997;8(2):i–viii.
57. Arvidsson A, Kokaia Z, Airaksinen M, Saarma M, Lindvall O. Stroke induces widespread changes of gene expression for glial cell line-derived neurotrophic factor family receptors in the adult rat brain. Neuroscience. 2001;106(1):27–41.
58. Krupinski J, Kumar P, Kumar S, Kaluza J. Increased expression of TGF-beta 1 in brain tissue after ischemic stroke in humans. Stroke. 1996;27(5):852–7.
59. Ausman JI, Ausman JI. Perioperative genomics. Surg Neurol. 2006;65(4):422.
60. Isbir SC, Tekeli A, Ergen A, Yilmaz H, Ak K, Civelek A, et al. Genetic polymorphisms contribute to acute kidney injury after coronary artery bypass grafting. Heart Surg Forum. 2007;10(6):E439–44.
61. Grigoryev DN, Liu M, Cheadle C, Barnes KC, Rabb H, Grigoryev DN, et al. Genomic profiling of kidney ischemia-reperfusion reveals expression of specific alloimmunity-associated genes: linking "immune" and "nonimmune" injury events. Transplant Proc. 2006;38(10):3333–6.
62. Rodrigo E, Sanchez-Velasco P, Ruiz JC, Fernandez-Fresnedo G, Lopez-Hoyos M, Pinera C, et al. Cytokine polymorphisms and risk of infection after kidney transplantation. Transplant Proc. 2007;39(7):2219–21.
63. Malik MH, Jury F, Bayat A, Ollier WE, Kay PR, Malik MHA, et al. Genetic susceptibility to total hip arthroplasty failure: a preliminary study on the influence of matrix metalloproteinase 1, interleukin 6 polymorphisms and vitamin D receptor. Ann Rheum Dis. 2007;66(8):1116–20.
64. Kolundzic R, Orlic D, Trkulja V, Pavelic K, Troselj KG, Kolundzic R, et al. Single nucleotide polymorphisms in the interleukin-6 gene promoter, tumor necrosis factor-alpha gene promoter, and transforming growth factor-beta1 gene signal sequence as predictors of time to onset of aseptic loosening after total hip arthroplasty: preliminary study. J Orthop Sci. 2006;11(6):592–600.
65. de Alvarenga MP, Pavarino-Bertelli EC, Abbud-Filho M, Ferreira-Baptista MA, Haddad R, Eberlin MN, et al. Combination of angiotensin-converting enzyme and methylenetetrahydrofolate reductase gene polymorphisms as determinant risk factors for chronic allograft dysfunction. Transplant Proc. 2007;39(1):78–80.

66. Sery O, Hrazdilova O, Didden W, Klenerova V, Staif R, Znojil V, et al. The association of monoamine oxidase B functional polymorphism with postoperative pain intensity. Neuro Endocrinol Lett. 2006;27(3):333–7.
67. Janicki PK, Schuler G, Francis D, Bohr A, Gordin V, Jarzembowski T, et al. A genetic association study of the functional A118G polymorphism of the human mu-opioid receptor gene in patients with acute and chronic pain. Anesth Analg. 2006;103(4):1011–7.
68. Kim H, Lee H, Rowan J, Brahim J, Dionne RA, Kim H, et al. Genetic polymorphisms in monoamine neurotransmitter systems show only weak association with acute post-surgical pain in humans. Mol Pain. 2006;2:24.
69. Chou WY, Yang LC, Lu HF, Ko JY, Wang CH, Lin SH, et al. Association of mu-opioid receptor gene polymorphism (A118G) with variations in morphine consumption for analgesia after total knee arthroplasty. Acta Anaesthesiol Scand. 2006;50(7):787–92.
70. Chou WY, Wang CH, Liu PH, Liu CC, Tseng CC, Jawan B, et al. Human opioid receptor A118G polymorphism affects intravenous patient-controlled analgesia morphine consumption after total abdominal hysterectomy. Anesthesiology. 2006;105(2):334–7 [see comment].
71. Bessler H, Shavit Y, Mayburd E, Smirnov G, Beilin B, Bessler H, et al. Postoperative pain, morphine consumption, and genetic polymorphism of IL-1beta and IL-1 receptor antagonist. Neurosci Lett. 2006;404(1–2):154–8.
72. Lee YS, Kim H, Wu TX, Wang XM, Dionne RA, Lee Y-S, et al. Genetically mediated interindividual variation in analgesic responses to cyclooxygenase inhibitory drugs. Clin Pharmacol Ther. 2006;79(5):407–18 [see comment].
73. Ryan R, Thornton J, Duggan E, McGovern E, O'Dwyer MJ, Ryan AW, et al. Gene polymorphism and requirement for vasopressor infusion after cardiac surgery. Ann Thorac Surg. 2006;82(3):895–901.
74. Podgoreanu MV, White WD, Morris RW, Mathew JP, Stafford-Smith M, Welsby IJ, et al. Inflammatory gene polymorphisms and risk of postoperative myocardial infarction after cardiac surgery. Circulation. 2006;114(1 Suppl):I275–81.
75. Bittar MN, Carey JA, Barnard JB, Pravica V, Deiraniya AK, Yonan N, et al. Tumor necrosis factor alpha influences the inflammatory response after coronary surgery. Ann Thorac Surg. 2006;81(1):132–7 [see comment].
76. Miriuka SG, Langman LJ, Evrovski J, Miner SE, Kozuszko S, D'Mello N, et al. Thromboembolism in heart transplantation: role of prothrombin G20210A and factor V Leiden. Transplantation. 2005;80(5):590–4.
77. Ozbek N, Atac FB, Yildirim SV, Verdi H, Yazici C, Yilmaz BT, et al. Analysis of prothrombotic mutations and polymorphisms in children who developed thrombosis in the perioperative period of congenital cardiac surgery. Cardiol Young. 2005;15(1):19–25.
78. Grocott HP, White WD, Morris RW, Podgoreanu MV, Mathew JP, Nielsen DM, et al. Genetic polymorphisms and the risk of stroke after cardiac surgery. Stroke. 2005;36(9):1854–8.
79. Unno N, Nakamura T, Mitsuoka H, Saito T, Miki K, Ishimaru K, et al. Single nucleotide polymorphism (G994—>T) in the plasma platelet-activating factor-acetylhydrolase gene is associated with graft patency of femoropopliteal bypass. Surgery. 2002;132(1):66–71.
80. Walter DH, Schachinger V, Elsner M, Mach S, Dimmeler S, Auch-Schwelk W, et al. Statin therapy is associated with reduced restenosis rates after coronary stent implantation in carriers of the Pl(A2)allele of the platelet glycoprotein IIIa gene. Eur Heart J. 2001;22(7):587–95 [see comment].
81. O'Hara AM, Shanahan F. The gut flora as a forgotten organ. EMBO Rep. 2006;7(7):688–93.
82. Round JL, Mazmanian SK. The gut microbiota shapes intestinal immune responses during health and disease. Nat Rev Immunol. 2009;9(5):313–23.
83. Fox AC, McConnell KW, Yoseph BP, Breed E, Liang Z, Clark AT, et al. The endogenous bacteria alter gut epithelial apoptosis and decrease mortality following pseudomonas aeruginosa pneumonia. Shock. 2012;38(5):508–14.
84. Fagundes CT, Amaral FA, Vieira AT, Soares AC, Pinho V, Nicoli JR, et al. Transient TLR activation restores inflammatory response and ability to control pulmonary bacterial infection in germfree mice. J Immunol. 2012;188(3):1411–20.

85. Mittal R, Coopersmith CM. Redefining the gut as the motor of critical illness. Trends Mol Med. 2014;20(4):214–23.

86. Babrowski T, Romanowski K, Fink D, Kim M, Gopalakrishnan V, Zaborina O, et al. The intestinal environment of surgical injury transforms Pseudomonas aeruginosa into a discrete hypervirulent morphotype capable of causing lethal peritonitis. Surgery. 2013;153(1):36–43.

87. Romanowski K, Zaborin A, Valuckaite V, Rolfes RJ, Babrowski T, Bethel C, et al. Candida albicans isolates from the gut of critically ill patients respond to phosphate limitation by expressing filaments and a lethal phenotype. PLoS One. 2012;7(1):e30119.

88. Khailova L, Frank DN, Dominguez JA, Wischmeyer PE. Probiotic administration reduces mortality and improves intestinal epithelial homeostasis in experimental sepsis. Anesthesiology. 2013;119(1):166–77.

89. Shimizu K, Ogura H, Asahara T, Nomoto K, Morotomi M, Tasaki O, et al. Probiotic/synbiotic therapy for treating critically Ill patients from a gut microbiota perspective. Dig Dis Sci. 2013;58(1):23–32.

90. Gennai S, Monsel A, Hao Q, Liu J, Gudapati V, Barbier EL, et al. Cell-based therapy for traumatic brain injury. Br J Anaesth. 2015;115(2):203–12.

91. Lee JS, Hong JM, Moon GJ, Lee PH, Ahn YH, Bang OY, et al. A long-term follow-up study of intravenous autologous mesenchymal stem cell transplantation in patients with ischemic stroke. Stem Cells. 2010;28(6):1099–106.

92. Pang X, Yang H, Peng B. Human umbilical cord mesenchymal stem cell transplantation for the treatment of chronic discogenic low back pain. Pain Physician. 2014;17(4):E525–30.

93. Dubois MJ, Vincent JL. Clinically-oriented therapies in sepsis: a review. J Endotoxin Res. 2000;6(6):463–9.

94. Eichacker PQ, Parent C, Kalil A, Esposito C, Cui X, Banks SM, et al. Risk and the efficacy of antiinflammatory agents: retrospective and confirmatory studies of sepsis. Am J Respir Crit Care Med. 2002;166(9):1197–205.

95. Vincent JL, Sun Q, Dubois MJ. Clinical trials of immunomodulatory therapies in severe sepsis and septic shock. Clin Infect Dis. 2002;34(8):1084–93.

96. Harris HW, Grunfeld C, Feingold KR, Read TE, Kane JP, Jones AL, et al. Chylomicrons alter the fate of endotoxin, decreasing tumor necrosis factor release and preventing death. J Clin Invest. 1993;91(3):1028–34.

97. Lanza-Jacoby S, Miller S, Jacob S, Heumann D, Minchenko AG, Flynn JT. Hyperlipoproteinemic low-density lipoprotein receptor-deficient mice are more susceptible to sepsis than corresponding wild-type mice. J Endotoxin Res. 2003;9(6):341–7.

98. Walley KR, Thain KR, Russell JA, Reilly MP, Meyer NJ, Ferguson JF, et al. PCSK9 is a critical regulator of the innate immune response and septic shock outcome. Sci Transl Med. 2014;6(258):258ra143.

99. László I, Trásy D, Molnár Z, Fazakas J. Sepsis: from pathophysiology to individualized patient care. J Immunol Res. 2015;2015.

100. Strober W, Fuss IJ. Proinflammatory cytokines in the pathogenesis of inflammatory bowel diseases. Gastroenterology. 2011;140(6):1756–67.

101. Bentzer P, Russell JA, Walley KR. Advances in sepsis research. Clin Chest Med. 2015;36(3):521–30.

102. Vincent JL, De Backer D. Circulatory shock. N Engl J Med. 2013;369(18):1726–34.

103. Dellinger RP, Levy MM, Rhodes A, Annane D, Gerlach H, Opal SM, et al. Surviving sepsis campaign: international guidelines for management of severe sepsis and septic shock: 2012. Crit Care Med. 2013;41(2):580–637.

104. Dubniks M, Persson J, Grände PO. Effect of blood pressure on plasma volume loss in the rat under increased permeability. Intensive Care Med. 2007;33(12):2192–8.

105. Nygren A, Redfors B, ThorÉn A, Ricksten SE. Norepinephrine causes a pressure-dependent plasma volume decrease in clinical vasodilatory shock. Acta Anaesthesiol Scand. 2010;54(7):814–20.

106. Rehberg S, Ertmer C, Vincent JL, Morelli A, Schneider M, Lange M, et al. Role of selective V1a receptor agonism in ovine septic shock. Crit Care Med. 2011;39(1):119–25.
107. Maybauer MO, Maybauer DM, Enkhbaatar P, Laporte R, Winiewska H, Traber LD, et al. The selective vasopressin type 1a receptor agonist selepressin (FE 202158) blocks vascular leak in ovine severe sepsis. Crit Care Med. 2014;42(7):e525–33.
108. Peng X, Hassoun PM, Sammani S, McVerry BJ, Burne MJ, Rabb H, et al. Protective effects of sphingosine 1-phosphate in murine endotoxin-induced inflammatory lung injury. Am J Respir Crit Care Med. 2004;169(11):1245–51.
109. Lundblad C, Axelberg H, Grände PO. Treatment with the sphingosine-1-phosphate analogue FTY 720 reduces loss of plasma volume during experimental sepsis in the rat. Acta Anaesthesiol Scand. 2013;57(6):713–8.
110. Wang L, Sammani S, Moreno-Vinasco L, Letsiou E, Wang T, Camp SM, et al. FTY720 (S)-phosphonate preserves sphingosine 1-phosphate receptor 1 expression and Exhibits superior barrier protection to FTY720 in acute lung injury. Crit Care Med. 2014;42(3):e189–99.
111. Wang Z, Sims CR, Patil NK, Gokden N, Mayeux PR. Pharmacologic targeting of sphingosine-1-phosphate receptor 1 improves the renal microcirculation during sepsis in the mouse. J Pharmacol Exp Ther. 2015;352(1):61–6.
112. Kumaraswamy SB, Linder A, Åkesson P, Dahlbäck B. Decreased plasma concentrations of apolipoprotein M in sepsis and systemic inflammatory response syndromes. Crit Care. 2012;16(2):R60.
113. Talmor DS, Fessler HE. Are esophageal pressure measurements important in clinical decision-making in mechanically ventilated patients? Respir Care. 2010;55(2):162–72.
114. Fan E, Needham DM, Stewart TE. Ventilatory management of acute lung injury and acute respiratory distress syndrome. JAMA. 2005;294(22):2889–96.
115. Putensen C, Theuerkauf N, Zinserling J, Wrigge H, Pelosi P. Meta-analysis: ventilation strategies and outcomes of the acute respiratory distress syndrome and acute lung injury. Ann Intern Med. 2009;151(8):566–76.
116. Petrucci N, Iacovelli W. Lung protective ventilation strategy for the acute respiratory distress syndrome. Cochrane Database Syst Rev. 2007;3.
117. Petrucci N, De Feo C. Lung protective ventilation strategy for the acute respiratory distress syndrome. Cochrane Database Syst Rev. 2013;2, CD003844.
118. Hager DN, Brower RG. Customizing lung-protective mechanical ventilation strategies. Crit Care Med. 2006;34(5):1554–5.
119. Talmor D, Sarge T, Malhotra A, O'Donnell CR, Ritz R, Lisbon A, et al. Mechanical ventilation guided by esophageal pressure in acute lung injury. N Engl J Med. 2008;359(20):2095–104.
120. Fish E, Novack V, Banner-Goodspeed VM, Sarge T, Loring S, Talmor D. The Esophageal Pressure-Guided Ventilation 2 (EPVent2) trial protocol: a multicentre, randomised clinical trial of mechanical ventilation guided by transpulmonary pressure. BMJ Open. 2014;4(9):e006356.
121. Amato MBP, Meade MO, Slutsky AS, Brochard L, Costa ELV, Schoenfeld DA, et al. Driving pressure and survival in the acute respiratory distress syndrome. N Engl J Med. 2015;372(8):747–55.
122. Forel JM, Roch A, Marin V, Michelet P, Demory D, Blache JL, et al. Neuromuscular blocking agents decrease inflammatory response in patients presenting with acute respiratory distress syndrome. Crit Care Med. 2006;34(11):2749–57.
123. Papazian L, Forel JM, Gacouin A, Penot-Ragon C, Perrin G, Loundou A, et al. Neuromuscular blockers in early acute respiratory distress syndrome. N Engl J Med. 2010;363(12):1107–16.
124. Gattinoni LG, Tognoni G, Pesenti A, Taccone P, Mascheroni D, Labarta V, et al. Effect of prone positioning on the survival of patients with acute respiratory failure. N Engl J Med. 2001;345(8):568–73.

125. Mancebo J, Fernández R, Blanch L, Rialp G, Gordo F, Ferrer M, et al. A multicenter trial of prolonged prone ventilation in severe acute respiratory distress syndrome. Am J Respir Crit Care Med. 2006;173(11):1233–9.
126. Guérin C, Reignier J, Richard JC, Beuret P, Gacouin A, Boulain T, et al. Prone positioning in severe acute respiratory distress syndrome. N Engl J Med. 2013;368(23):2159–68.
127. Hager DN. Recent advances in the management of the acute respiratory distress syndrome. Clin Chest Med. 2015;36(3):481–96.
128. Henzler D, Mahnken AH, Wildberger JE, Rossaint R, Günther RW, Kuhlen R. Multislice spiral computed tomography to determine the effects of a recruitment maneuver in experimental lung injury. Eur Radiol. 2006;16(6):1351–9.
129. Pelosi P, Rocco PR, De Abreu MG. Use of computed tomography scanning to guide lung recruitment and adjust positive-end expiratory pressure. Curr Opin Crit Care. 2011;17(3):268–74.
130. Frerichs I, Hinz J, Herrmann P, Weisser G, Hahn G, Dudykevych T, et al. Detection of local lung air content by electrical impedance tomography compared with electron beam CT. J Appl Physiol. 2002;93(2):660–6.
131. Victorino JA, Borges JB, Okamoto VN, Matos GFJ, Tucci MR, Caramez MPR, et al. Imbalances in regional lung ventilation: a validation study on electrical impedance tomography. Am J Respir Crit Care Med. 2004;169(7):791–800.
132. Meier T, Luepschen H, Karsten J, Leibecke T, Großherr M, Gehring H, et al. Assessment of regional lung recruitment and derecruitment during a PEEP trial based on electrical impedance tomography. Intensive Care Med. 2008;34(3):543–50.
133. Wrigge H, Zinserling J, Muders T, Varelmann D, Günther U, Von Der Groeben C, et al. Electrical impedance tomography compared with thoracic computed tomography during a slow inflation maneuver in experimental models of lung injury. Crit Care Med. 2008;36(3):903–9.
134. Frerichs I, Dargaville PA, Van Genderingen H, Morel DR, Rimensberger PC. Lung volume recruitment after surfactant administration modifies spatial distribution of ventilation. Am J Respir Crit Care Med. 2006;174(7):772–9.
135. Zhao Z, Möller K, Steinmann D, Frerichs I, Guttmann J. Evaluation of an electrical impedance tomography-based global inhomogeneity index for pulmonary ventilation distribution. Intensive Care Med. 2009;35(11):1900–6.
136. Blankman P, Hasan D, Erik GJ, Gommers D. Detection of 'best' positive end-expiratory pressure derived from electrical impedance tomography parameters during a decremental positive end-expiratory pressure trial. Crit Care. 2014;18(3):R95.
137. Hypothermia_After_Cardiac_Arrest_Study_Group. Mild therapeutic hypothermia to improve the neurologic outcome after cardiac arrest. N Engl J Med. 2002;346(8):549–56.
138. Bernard S, Gray T, Buist M, Jones B, Silvester W, Gutteridge G, et al. Treatment of comatose survivors of out-of-hospital cardiac arrest with induced hypothermia. N Engl J Med. 2002;346(8):557–63.
139. Clifton G, Allen S, Barrodale P, Plenger P, Berry J, Koch S, et al. A phase II study of moderate hypothermia in severe brain injury. J Neurotrauma. 1993;10(3):263–71.
140. Marion D. Moderate hypothermia in severe head injuries: the present and the future. Curr Opin Crit Care. 2002;8(2):111–4.
141. Wypij D, Newburger J, Rappaport L, duPlessis A, Jonas R, Wernovsky G, et al. The effect of duration of deep hypothermic circulatory arrest in infant heart surgery on late neurodevelopment: the Boston Circulatory Arrest Trial. J Thorac Cardiovasc Surg. 2003;126(5):1397–403.
142. Augoustides JG, Floyd TF, McGarvey ML, Ochroch EA, Pochettino A, Fulford S, et al. Major clinical outcomes in adults undergoing thoracic aortic surgery requiring deep hypothermic circulatory arrest: quantification of organ-based perioperative outcome and detection of opportunities for perioperative intervention. J Cardiothorac Vasc Anesth. 2005;19(4):446–52.

143. Appoo JJ, Augoustides JG, Pochettino A, Savino JS, McGarvey ML, Cowie DC, et al. Perioperative outcome in adults undergoing elective deep hypothermic circulatory arrest with retrograde cerebral perfusion in proximal aortic arch repair: evaluation of protocol-based care. J Cardiothorac Vasc Anesth. 2006;20(1):3–7.
144. Drew KL, Buck CL, Barnes BM, Christian SL, Rasley BT, Harris MB, et al. Central nervous system regulation of mammalian hibernation: implications for metabolic suppression and ischemia tolerance. J Neurochem. 2007;102(6):1713–26.
145. Bellamy R, Safar P, Tisherman SA, Basford R, Bruttig SP, Capone A, et al. Suspended animation for delayed resuscitation. Crit Care Med. 1996;24(2 Suppl):S24–47.
146. Volpato GP, Searles R, Yu B, Scherrer-Crosbie M, Bloch KD, Ichinose F, et al. Inhaled hydrogen sulfide: a rapidly reversible inhibitor of cardiac and metabolic function in the mouse. Anesthesiology. 2008;108(4):659–68.
147. Andrews MT, Andrews MT. Advances in molecular biology of hibernation in mammals. Bioessays. 2007;29(5):431–40.
148. Wu X, Drabek T, Kochanek PM, Henchir J, Stezoski SW, Stezoski J, et al. Induction of profound hypothermia for emergency preservation and resuscitation allows intact survival after cardiac arrest resulting from prolonged lethal hemorrhage and trauma in dogs. Circulation. 2006;113(16):1974–82.
149. Tisherman SA, Tisherman SA. Hypothermia and injury. Curr Opin Crit Care. 2004;10(6):512–9.
150. Oron U, Ilic S, De Taboada L, Streeter J, Oron U, Ilic S, et al. Ga-As (808 nm) laser irradiation enhances ATP production in human neuronal cells in culture. Photomed Laser Surg. 2007;25(3):180–2.
151. Oron A, Oron U, Chen J, Eilam A, Zhang C, Sadeh M, et al. Low-level laser therapy applied transcranially to rats after induction of stroke significantly reduces long-term neurological deficits. Stroke. 2006;37(10):2620–4.
152. Detaboada L, Ilic S, Leichliter-Martha S, Oron U, Oron A, Streeter J, et al. Transcranial application of low-energy laser irradiation improves neurological deficits in rats following acute stroke. Lasers Surg Med. 2006;38(1):70–3.
153. Lapchak PA, Wei J, Zivin JA, Lapchak PA, Wei J, Zivin JA. Transcranial infrared laser therapy improves clinical rating scores after embolic strokes in rabbits. Stroke. 2004;35(8):1985–8.
154. Lampl Y, Zivin JA, Fisher M, Lew R, Welin L, Dahlof B, et al. Infrared laser therapy for ischemic stroke: a new treatment strategy: results of the NeuroThera Effectiveness and Safety Trial-1 (NEST-1). Stroke. 2007;38(6):1843–9.
155. Grotta J, Grotta J. Neuroprotection is unlikely to be effective in humans using current trial designs. Stroke. 2002;33(1):306–7 [see comment].
156. Medicine WUSo, NINDS, Association AS. Stroke Trials Registry St Louis 2008 [updated 4 Jan, 2008 7 Jan, 2008]. Available from: http://www.strokecenter.org/trials/index.aspx.
157. Donnan GA. The 2007 Feinberg lecture: a new road map for neuroprotection. Stroke. 2008;39(1):242.
158. Kofke WA. Incrementally applied multifaceted therapeutic bundles in neuroprotection clinical trials…time for change. Neurocrit Care. 2010;12(3):438–44.
159. Rossignol S, Schwab M, Schwartz M, Fehlings MG, Rossignol S, Schwab M, et al. Spinal cord injury: time to move? J Neurosci. 2007;27(44):11782–92.
160. Baptiste DC, Fehlings MG, Baptiste DC, Fehlings MG. Update on the treatment of spinal cord injury. Prog Brain Res. 2007;161:217–33.
161. Albin MS, White RJ, Acosta-Rua G, Yashon D, Albin MS, White RJ, et al. Study of functional recovery produced by delayed localized cooling after spinal cord injury in primates. J Neurosurg. 1968;29(2):113–20.
162. Albin MS, White RJ, Locke GS, Massopust Jr LC, Kretchmer HE, Albin MS, et al. Localized spinal cord hypothermia--anesthetic effects and application to spinal cord injury. Anesth Analg. 1967;46(1):8–16.

163. Albin MS, White RJ, Locke GE, Kretchmer HE, Albin MS, White RJ, et al. Spinal cord hypothermia by localized perfusion cooling. Nature. 1966;210(5040):1059–60.

164. Mesquita RC, D'Souza A, Bilfinger TV, Galler RM, Emanuel A, Schenkel SS, et al. Optical monitoring and detection of spinal cord ischemia. PLoS One. 2013;8:e83370.

165. McDonald JW, McDonald JW. Repairing the damaged spinal cord: from stem cells to activity-based restoration therapies. Clin Neurosurg. 2004;51:207–27.

166. McDonald JW, Howard MJ, McDonald JW, Howard MJ. Repairing the damaged spinal cord: a summary of our early success with embryonic stem cell transplantation and remyelination. Prog Brain Res. 2002;137:299–309.

167. Coutts M, Keirstead HS, Coutts M, Keirstead HS. Stem cells for the treatment of spinal cord injury. Exp Neurol. 2008;209(2):368–77.

168. Yoshihara T, Ohta M, Itokazu Y, Matsumoto N, Dezawa M, Suzuki Y, et al. Neuroprotective effect of bone marrow-derived mononuclear cells promoting functional recovery from spinal cord injury. J Neurotrauma. 2007;24(6):1026–36.

169. Tao X, Ming-Kun Y, Wei-Bin S, Hai-Long G, Rui K, Lai-Yong T. Role of telomerase reverse transcriptase in glial scar formation after spinal cord injury in rats. Neurochem Res. 2013;38(9):1914–20.

170. Genovese T, Mazzon E, Crisafulli C, Di Paola R, Muia C, Esposito E, et al. TNF-alpha blockage in a mouse model of SCI: evidence for improved outcome. Shock. 2008;29(1):32–41.

171. Zhang X, Zeng Y, Zhang W, Wang J, Wu J, Li J, et al. Co-transplantation of neural stem cells and NT-3-overexpressing Schwann cells in transected spinal cord. J Neurotrauma. 2007;24(12):1863–77.

172. Koda M, Kamada T, Hashimoto M, Murakami M, Shirasawa H, Sakao S, et al. Adenovirus vector-mediated ex vivo gene transfer of brain-derived neurotrophic factor to bone marrow stromal cells promotes axonal regeneration after transplantation in completely transected adult rat spinal cord. Eur Spine J. 2007;16(12):2206–14.

173. Biernaskie J, Sparling JS, Liu J, Shannon CP, Plemel JR, Xie Y, et al. Skin-derived precursors generate myelinating Schwann cells that promote remyelination and functional recovery after contusion spinal cord injury. J Neurosci. 2007;27(36):9545–59.

174. Boas D, Yodh A. Spatially varying dynamical properties of turbid media probed with diffusing temporal light correlation. J Opt Soc Am. 1997;14(1):192–215.

175. Cheung C, Culver JP, Takahashi K, Greenberg JH, Yodh AG. In vivo cerebrovascular measurement combining diffuse near-infrared absorption and correlation spectroscopies. Phys Med Biol. 2001;46(8):2053–65.

176. Boas DA, Campbell LE, Yodh AG. Scattering and imaging with diffusing temporal field correlations. Phys Rev Lett. 1995;75(9):1855–8.

177. Maret G, Wolf P. Multiple light scattering from disordered media, the effect of brownian motion of scatterers. Z Phys B Condens Matter. 1987;65(1):409–13.

178. Pine DJ, Weitz DA, Chaikin PM, Herbolzheimer E. Diffusing wave spectroscopy. Phys Rev Lett. 1988;60(12):1134–7.

179. Kim MN, Durduran T, Frangos S, Edlow BL, Buckley EM, Moss HE, et al. Noninvasive measurement of cerebral blood flow and blood oxygenation using near-infrared and diffuse correlation spectroscopies in critically brain-injured adults. Neurocrit Care. 2010;12(2):173–80.

180. Corlu A, Durduran T, Choe R, Schweiger M, Hillman EM, Arridge SR, et al. Uniqueness and wavelength optimization in continuous-wave multispectral diffuse optical tomography. Opt Lett. 2003;28(23):2339–41.

181. Corlu A, Choe R, Durduran T, Lee K, Schweiger M, Arridge SR, et al. Diffuse optical tomography with spectral constraints and wavelength optimization. Appl Opt. 2005;44(11):2082–93.

182. Chandra M, Balu R, Yodh A, Frangos S, Park S, Kofke W. Continuous Non-invasive measurement of cerebral blood flow metabolic rate for oxygen and oxygen extraction fraction in critically Ill brain injured patients. Neurocrit Care. 2014;12.

183. Schytz HW, Guo S, Jensen LT, Kamar M, Nini A, Gress DR, et al. A new technology for detecting cerebral blood flow: a comparative study of ultrasound tagged NIRS and 133Xe-SPECT. Neurocrit Care. 2012;17(1):139–45.
184. Schwarz M, Rivera G, Hammond M, Silman Z, Jackson K, Kofke WA. Acousto-optic cerebral blood flow monitoring during induction of anesthesia in humans. Neurocrit Care. 2015 Epub ahead of print.
185. Punjasawadwong Y, Boonjeungmonkol N, Phongchiewboon A, Punjasawadwong Y, Boonjeungmonkol N, Phongchiewboon A. Bispectral index for improving anaesthetic delivery and postoperative recovery. Cochrane Database Syst Rev. 2007;4, CD003843.
186. Bennett HL, Patel L, Farida N, Beddell S, Bobbin M. Separation of the hypnotic component of anesthesia and facial EMG responses to surgical stimulation. Anesthesiology. 2007;107:A730.
187. Gjerstad AC, Storm H, Hagen R, Huiku M, Qvigstad E, Raeder J, et al. Comparison of skin conductance with entropy during intubation, tetanic stimulation and emergence from general anaesthesia. Acta Anaesthesiol Scand. 2007;51(1):8–15.
188. Storm H, Shafiei M, Myre K, Raeder J, Storm H, Shafiei M, et al. Palmar skin conductance compared to a developed stress score and to noxious and awakening stimuli on patients in anaesthesia. Acta Anaesthesiol Scand. 2005;49(6):798–803.
189. Larson MD, Kurz A, Sessler DI, Dechert M, Bjorksten AR, Tayefeh F, et al. Alfentanil blocks reflex pupillary dilation in response to noxious stimulation but does not diminish the light reflex. Anesthesiology. 1997;87(4):849–55.
190. Hemmerling TM, Salhab E, Aoun G, Charabati S, Mathieu PA, editors. The 'Analgoscore': a novel score to monitor intraoperative pain and its use for remifentanil closed-loop application. 2007 IEEE International Conference on Systems, Man, and Cybernetics, SMC 2007; Montreal; 2007.
191. Hemmerling TM, Arbeid E, Wehbe M, Cyr S, Taddei R, Zaouter C, et al. Evaluation of a novel closed-loop total intravenous anaesthesia drug delivery system: A randomized controlled trial. Br J Anaesth. 2013;110(6):1031–9.
192. Wehbe M, Arbeid E, Cyr S, Mathieu PA, Taddei R, Morse J, et al. A technical description of a novel pharmacological anesthesia robot. J Clin Monit Comput. 2014;28(1):27–34.
193. Hemmerling TM, Taddei R, Wehbe M, Zaouter C, Cyr S, Morse J. First robotic tracheal intubations in humans using the Kepler intubation system. Br J Anaesth. 2012;108(6):1011–6.
194. Hemmerling TM, Wehbe M, Zaouter C, Taddei R, Morse J. The kepler intubation system. Anesth Analg. 2012;114(3):590–4.
195. Firlik AD, Kaufmann AM, Wechsler LR, Firlik KS, Fukui MB, Yonas H. Quantitative cerebral blood flow determinations in acute ischemic stroke: relationship to computed tomography and angiography. Stroke. 1997;28(11):2208–13.
196. Firlik AD, Rubin G, Yonas H, Wechsler LR. Relation between cerebral blood flow and neurologic deficit resolution in acute ischemic stroke. Neurology. 1998;51(1):177–82.
197. Rubin G, Firlik AD, Levy EI, Pindzola RR, Yonas H. Relationship between cerebral blood flow and clinical outcome in acute stroke. Cerebrovasc Dis. 2000;10(4):298–306.
198. Stiefel M, Spiotta A, Gracias V, Garuffe A, Guillamondegui O, Maloney-Wilensky E, et al. Reduced mortality rate in patients with severe traumatic brain injury treated with brain tissue oxygen monitoring. J Neurosurg. 2005;103(5):805–11.
199. Bellander B-M, Cantais E, Enblad P, Hutchinson P, Nordstrom C-H, Robertson C, et al. Consensus meeting on microdialysis in neurointensive care. Intensive Care Med. 2004;30(12):2166–9.
200. Sarrafzadeh A, Haux D, Sakowitz O, Benndorf G, Herzog H, Kuechler I, et al. Acute focal neurological deficits in aneurysmal subarachnoid hemorrhage: relation of clinical course, CT findings, and metabolite abnormalities monitored with bedside microdialysis. Stroke. 2003;34(6):1382–8.

201. Sarrafzadeh AS, Haux D, Ludemann L, Amthauer H, Plotkin M, Kuchler I, et al. Cerebral ischemia in aneurysmal subarachnoid hemorrhage: a correlative microdialysis-PET study. Stroke. 2004;35(3):638–43.

202. Le Roux P, Menon DK, Citerio G, Vespa P, Bader MK, Brophy GM, et al. Consensus summary statement of the international multidisciplinary consensus conference on multimodality monitoring in neurocritical care: a statement for healthcare professionals from the neurocritical care society and the european society of intensive care medicine. Intensive Care Med. 2014;40(9):1189–209.

203. Thaler ER, Hanson CW, Thaler ER, Hanson CW. Medical applications of electronic nose technology. Expert Rev Med Devices. 2005;2(5):559–66.

204. Hockstein NG, Thaler ER, Lin Y, Lee DD, Hanson CW, Hockstein NG, et al. Correlation of pneumonia score with electronic nose signature: a prospective study. Ann Otol Rhinol Laryngol. 2005;114(7):504–8.

205. Thaler ER, Hanson CW, Thaler ER, Hanson CW. Use of an electronic nose to diagnose bacterial sinusitis. Am J Rhinol. 2006;20(2):170–2.

206. Dragonieri S, Schot R, Mertens BJ, Le Cessie S, Gauw SA, Spanevello A, et al. An electronic nose in the discrimination of patients with asthma and controls. J Allergy Clin Immunol. 2007;120(4):856–62.

207. Gendron KB, Hockstein NG, Thaler ER, Vachani A, Hanson CW, Gendron KB, et al. In vitro discrimination of tumor cell lines with an electronic nose. Otolaryngol Head Neck Surg. 2007;137(2):269–73.

208. Anonymous. Electronic nose shows promise for detecting early-stage lung cancer. Dis Manag Advis. 2005;11(6):71–2.

209. Fend R, Kolk AH, Bessant C, Buijtels P, Klatser PR, Woodman AC, et al. Prospects for clinical application of electronic-nose technology to early detection of Mycobacterium tuberculosis in culture and sputum. J Clin Microbiol. 2006;44(6):2039–45.

210. Olsen E, Vogt G, Ekeberg D, Sandbakk M, Pettersen J, Nilsson A, et al. Analysis of the early stages of lipid oxidation in freeze-stored pork back fat and mechanically recovered poultry meat. J Agric Food Chem. 2005;53(2):338–48.

211. Behn C, Araneda OF, Llanos AJ, Celedon G, Gonzalez G, Behn C, et al. Hypoxia-related lipid peroxidation: evidences, implications and approaches. Respir Physiol Neurobiol. 2007;158(2–3):143–50.

212. Muralikrishna Adibhatla R, Hatcher JF, Muralikrishna Adibhatla R, Hatcher JF. Phospholipase A2, reactive oxygen species, and lipid peroxidation in cerebral ischemia. Free Radic Biol Med. 2006;40(3):376–87.

213. Warner DS, Sheng H, Batinic-Haberle I, Warner DS, Sheng H, Batinic-Haberle I. Oxidants, antioxidants and the ischemic brain. J Exp Biol. 2004;207(Pt 18):3221–31.

214. Salvemini D, Cuzzocrea S, Salvemini D, Cuzzocrea S. Superoxide, superoxide dismutase and ischemic injury. Curr Opin Investig Drugs. 2002;3(6):886–95.

215. Vespa PM, Vespa PM. Multimodality monitoring and telemonitoring in neurocritical care: from microdialysis to robotic telepresence. Curr Opin Crit Care. 2005;11(2):133–8.

216. Breslow M, Rosenfeld B, Doerfler M, Burke G, Yates G, Stone D, et al. Effect of a multiple-site intensive care unit telemedicine program on clinical and economic outcomes: an alternative paradigm for intensivist staffing. Crit Care Med. 2004;32(1):31–8.

217. Celi L, et al. The eICU; It's not just telemedicine. Crit Care Med. 2001;29(8):N183.

218. Friedman EB, Sun Y, Moore JT, Hung H, Meng QC, Perera P, et al. A conserved behavioral state barrier impedes transitions between anesthetic-induced unconsciousness and wakefulness: evidence for neural inertia. PLoS One. 2010;5(7):e11903.

219. Joiner WJ, Friedman EB, Hung HT, Koh K, Sowcik M, Sehgal A, et al. Genetic and anatomical basis of the barrier separating wakefulness and anesthetic-induced unresponsiveness. PLoS Genet. 2013;9(9):e1003605.

220. Kelz MB, Sun Y, Chen J, Cheng Meng Q, Moore JT, Veasey SC, et al. An essential role for orexins in emergence from general anesthesia. Proc Natl Acad Sci U S A. 2008;105(4):1309–14.
221. Antonik LJ, Goldwater DR, Kilpatrick GJ, Tilbrook GS, Borkett KM. A placebo-and midazolam-controlled phase i single ascending-dose study evaluating the safety, pharmacokinetics, and pharmacodynamics of remimazolam (CNS 7056): part I. Safety, efficacy, and basic pharmacokinetics. Anesth Analg. 2012;115(2):274–83.
222. Worthington MT, Antonik LJ, Goldwater DR, Lees JP, Wilhelm-Ogunbiyi K, Borkett KM, et al. A phase ib, dose-finding study of multiple doses of remimazolam (cns 7056) in volunteers undergoing colonoscopy. Anesth Analg. 2013;117(5):1093–100.

Chapter 16
Health Care in the Year 2050 and Beyond

Brian Wowk

> *"It is the great glory as well as the great threat of science that everything which is in principle possible can be done if the intention to do it is sufficiently resolute".*
>
> Sir Peter Medawar

Four decades is a long time. In 1927 Charles Lindbergh flew from New York to Paris in 33 hours. 1969 saw the first flight of the supersonic Concorde, which would carry 100 passengers over the Atlantic ten times faster at the edge of space. In 1970 the PDP-11 with 56 kilobytes memory was a popular business computer. In 2011 a pocket smartphone can have a million times more memory.

Sometimes four decades is less significant. Although there have been improvements in safety and economy, the speed of commercial air travel has not increased since 1970. Our computers may be a million times more powerful, but we are not a million times smarter, a million times wealthier, or living a million times longer. Technology may even be breeding a sedentary shorter-lived generation accustomed to having information at their fingertips rather than knowledge in their head. There can be big disconnects between technology and outcomes.

New medical technology is sharply restrained by social factors. Low tolerance for adverse outcomes and associated heavy regulation limit the pace of innovation compared to other fields. What is possible is by no means what will necessarily be done.

Nevertheless, in contemplating health care in 2050, we must be open to the possibility that medicine might become something almost unrecognizable to us today. Historical developments such as vaccines and anesthesia can and have fundamentally changed medicine and public health. Developments of similar magnitude are possible over the next half century. Medicine still operates far from the bounds of what is possible according to known physical law.

B. Wowk, PhD
21st Century Medicine, Inc., Fontana, CA, USA
e-mail: wowk@21cm.com

© Springer International Publishing Switzerland 2016   147
D. Crippen (ed.), *The Intensivist's Challenge: Aging and Career Growth in a High-Stress Medical Specialty*, DOI 10.1007/978-3-319-30454-0_16

In attempting to visualize what may come, it is helpful to view health care in three parts: information, intelligence, and intervention. There is information about health, the process of deciding what to do about it, and what interventions by way of prevention or therapy are available. All three parts will see great change in coming decades.

Information

We are in the midst of an explosion of information. The explosion is driven by both new diagnostic methods and information processing/communication systems. The component density and information storage capacity of computers has been doubling every 2 years since the 1960s (Moore's Law) (Fig. 16.1). Processing speed has also been increasing exponentially (Fig. 16.2).

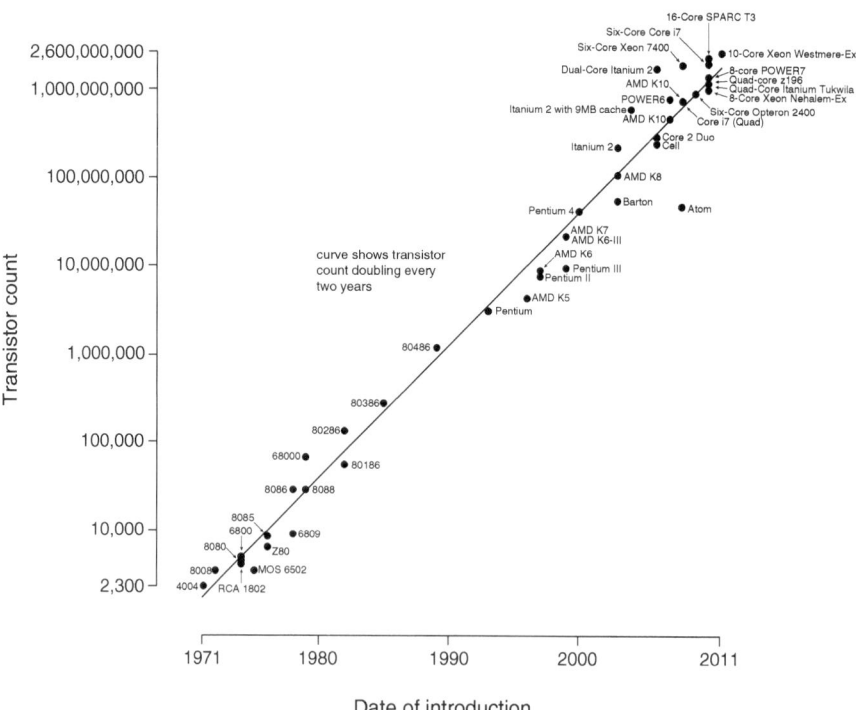

Fig. 16.1 Computer microprocessor transistor counts as a function of year (Image by Wikipedia user Wgsimon, CC BY-SA 3.0 license)

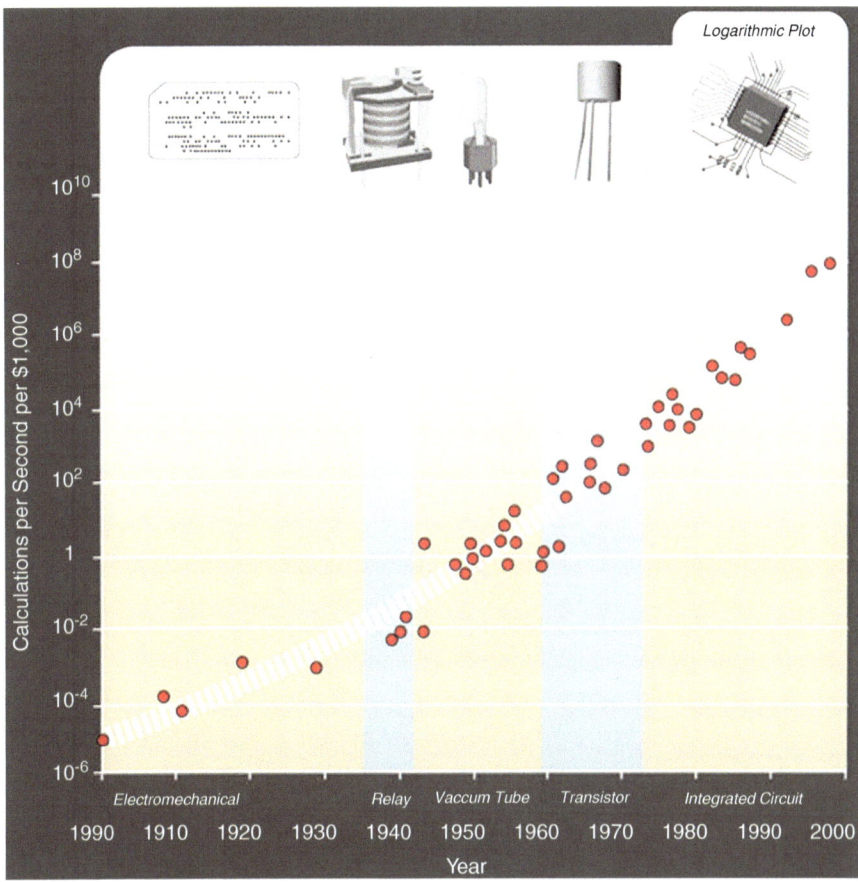

Fig. 16.2 Computer processor speed as a function of year (Image adapted from Ray Kurzweil and Kurzweil Technologies, Inc., CC BY 1.0 license)

These trends are projected to end circa 2018 as present chip fabrication methods hit physical limits. However, other technologies such as three-dimensional fabrication, molecular electronics, and nanotechnology are waiting in the wings to continue miniaturization trends for perhaps several more decades. The use of small molecules or individual atoms as information storage elements would seem to be the ultimate physical limit for computer miniaturization, a limit to be reached later this century. In the mid-twenty-first century, mere cubic centimeters can be expected to hold 1000 terabytes of information and parallel processors capable of executing 10^{15} instructions per second. This is the information processing capacity of ten human brains contained in a small electronic device.

This capacity will not go unused. Diagnostic information is undergoing its own exponential increase. The cost of completely sequencing a human genome, approximately one billion US dollars in the 1990s, is now plummeting toward

$1,000 and lower [1] (Fig. 16.3). By 2025 a patient's genome will be part of their medical record, to eventually be joined by their epigenome, proteome, and transcriptome of multiple cell types. The latter parameters of systems biology will be measured with greater frequency and utility as measurement costs continue declining and understanding of their meaning increases.

"Lab on a chip" miniaturization will decrease the cost and infrastructure required for clinical laboratory tests, moving them to the point of care. Just as photography no longer requires film processing labs, diagnostic tests may no longer require clinical laboratories. Microfluidic laboratories will track numerous biomarkers, analyze circulating cells, and even determine the transcriptome of cells. Cancer will be detected at the earliest stages. Inflammation status will be known in detail, including whether the cause of inflammation is disease, trauma, or pathogens. Real-time PCR and other on-chip technologies will permit detection and identification of pathogens on timescales of minutes [2]. By the mid-twenty-first century, these analytical capabilities will be available in very small packages.

Miniaturization of other diagnostic and monitoring technology continues apace. Pill cameras transmitting GI tract images are already a reality. The smallest ultrasound scanner in 2011 is a handheld wand connected to a smartphone [3]. Cardiac monitoring systems with long-term data recording and telemetry will soon be completely unobtrusive. Instrumentation and telemetry of chronically ill patients will contribute to the deluge of information available to physicians. Low cost and

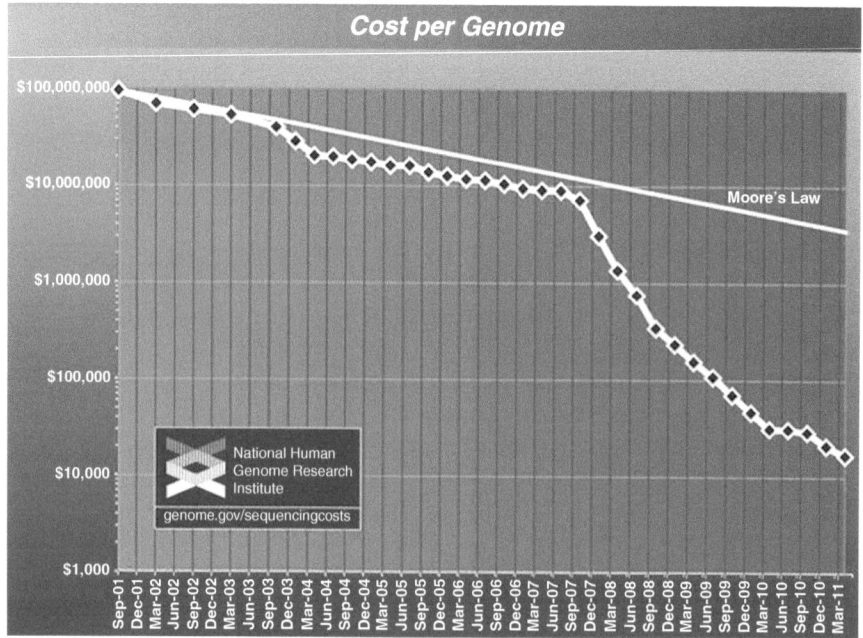

Fig. 16.3 Cost for sequencing an entire human genome (Image from National Human Genome Research Institute)

unobtrusiveness will lead to greater adoption of personal medical monitoring technologies by the healthy, with or without physician involvement. Some of this technology may be surgically implanted. Many people today elect to have surgical implants for reasons of vanity. In the mid-twenty-first century, implants providing detailed personal health monitoring may be popular (Fig. 16.4).

In the fictional television show "Star Trek," doctors diagnosed by waving a small "tricorder" over a patient. In 2050 real diagnostics may consist of physicians or EMS personnel reading a small device held near a patient, receiving wireless telemetry of vital signs, clinical chemistries, and real-time molecular diagnostics from permanently implanted sensors. Power and substrate for analytical processes might be derived entirely in vivo.

Intelligence

With thousands of measured parameters, and even the patient's entire genome added to the mix, automated processing of diagnostic information will be a vital element of twenty-first century medicine. Computers will digest torrents of information into smaller streams of what is most clinically relevant. Raw measurements will be fed into sophisticated models of cell and organism physiology, drawing upon worldwide biomedical databases to construct the clinical picture of an individual patient.

Clinical decision support systems with computerized physician order entry are already part of medicine. Some of these systems generate automated medication selection and dose recommendations. With increasing complexity of the critical care environment, automation of dosing and administration based on process control feedback is foreseeable. In time-sensitive settings, physicians have already ceded

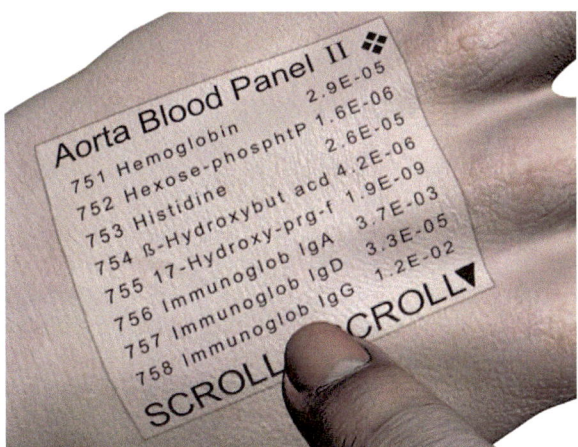

Fig. 16.4 Personal health monitoring in 2050? A dermal thin film display shows readings from implanted sensors (Concept by Robert Freitas. Artwork by Gina Miller © www.nanogirl.com)

dramatic interventions to automated systems. Implantable cardioverter-defibrillators are an example. The work of the critical care physician of the future may be analogous to that of a modern airline pilot giving direction to automation systems. Most of the flight time of modern airliners is not spent under the direct control of pilots.

Technology will allow the human intelligence of medicine to extend its reach. "eICU" telemedicine systems are already making inroads into critical care. Physicians using the RP-7 robotic telepresence system have run cardiac arrests from home [4]. Information will be also accessible to physicians via their personal computing and communication devices. In 2011 the US FDA approved the first app for image reading and mobile diagnoses by radiologists using the Apple iPhone and iPad [5]. On the patient side, the same personal monitoring technologies that would allow point-of-care "tricorder" readings of vital signs and clinical chemistries could be configured for remote telemetry via a patient's personal communication device. Some remote interventions will also be possible, such as adjustment of implanted therapeutic devices.

It is difficult to predict just how much human intelligence will be replaceable by computers in 2050. Early predictions of the progress of artificial intelligence (AI) made in the 1960s have not come to pass even though the world's most powerful computers now exceed the processing capacity of the human brain. Such capacity will exist on the desktop by 2025. However, human information processing capacity does not necessarily equal human intelligence.

Nowadays AI means expert systems adept at specialized information processing. The original aspiration of AI, the creation of humanlike general intelligence in computers, is now called AGI (artificial general intelligence). A few small groups still pursue this objective, with the creation of computer programs capable of self-improvement viewed as an especially important milestone. A general intelligence capable of understanding and improving itself could theoretically lead to the rapid growth of entities with intelligence far greater than the human mind. This hypothetical development has been termed "the singularity." The timing and effects of such a development remain controversial.

In 2011 chat bots are able to pass superficial Turing tests. Engines able to search the Internet and other deep databases using natural conversational language will be a reality by 2020 if not sooner. A powerful IBM computer named "Watson" beat the best human contestants in the American trivia quiz show, "Jeopardy," in 2011. Watson was designed to be an AI physician and has begun demonstrations in that role [6]. Watson's ability to rapidly digest electronic health records and analyze diagnostic images is expected to make radiology an especially fruitful role [7].

Conservatively, we can predict that by 2050 expert systems will exist that permit patients to discuss medical issues with computers using natural language. For health-care professionals, computers with access to deep databases of medical records, journal articles, references works, and models of physiology will be able to engage in sophisticated conversation about patients and treatment plans. Medicine will become a partnership between physician, patient, and machine.

Intervention

The dramatic advances underway in the information and intelligence of medicine are driven by advances in the unregulated and highly competitive fields of computer software and microelectronics. Intervention is a different story. The number of new drugs (new molecular entities) brought to market per year has been flat since 1940, averaging about 20 a year in the USA [8]. Worse, the productivity of pharmaceutical research has been exponentially *decreasing*. Since the 1962 Kefauver Amendment to the US Food, Drug, and Cosmetic Act, the inflation-adjusted R&D cost to bring a new drug to market has doubled every 7.5 years in a sort of Moore's Law in reverse [8]. Entire market sectors are being abandoned by pharmaceutical companies because they cannot afford the contemporary costs of drug development. There are some hopeful signs that the productivity decline may have bottomed out in 2006 [9]. Nevertheless, the present cost and regulatory burden of new drug development makes optimism about treatment progress via the traditional pharmaceutical development pipeline difficult. The days of medical device "hackers" like Walton Lillehei or Willem Kolff inventing new forms of life support in small shops with small budgets are also long gone.

Sociopolitical and business realities aside, the scientific prospects for new disease treatments and cures during the twenty-first century are bright. Detailed understanding of molecular pathways of disease and health will facilitate the development of biologics with greater therapeutic reach than mere enzyme or receptor-binding agents. Regenerative medicine will rebuild damaged or defective tissue. Eventually the ability to build and control systems on the molecular scale will profoundly change the nature of medicine itself.

Interventions facilitated by continuing advances in electronics technology are easiest to predict. Surgery will continue to become less invasive as technology permits surgeons to do more work with their hands outside the patient. Microrobotic telepresence will open new frontiers of surgery. Natural orifice transluminal endoscopic surgery will permit some surgeries to be done without ever cutting skin. Brain-computer interface (BCI) technology will lead to prosthetic limb replacements that patients move and feel like their own limbs. Artificial retinas will advance in the twenty-first century as cochlear implants did in the twentieth. Noncortical blindness will be curable.

In the longer term, electronic fixes for sensory or motor deficits are just expensive stop-gap measures. Regenerative medicine, comprising injection of stem cells, transplantation of engineered tissue and organs, and induced regeneration of tissue, organs, and limbs will eventually render prosthetic devices obsolete. A possible exception may be devices that do more than biology can, such as implanted communication/computing devices interfaced directly to the brain. Routine use of such devices is possible by 2050.

Patients with artery disease may be among the early beneficiaries of regenerative medicine. Bone-marrow-derived endothelial progenitor cells (EPCs) play a pivotal role in maintenance of vascular endothelium. There is evidence that EPCs prevent and even reverse the damage of atherosclerosis [10]. By the middle of this century, infusion of EPCs derived from rejuvenated pluripotent stem cells may be able to restore a patient's entire vascular endothelium to a youthful state. This one intervention could at once cure heart disease, cerebrovascular disease, and peripheral artery disease and prevent at least some forms of dementia.

By the mid-twenty-first century, cancer should be comprehensively curable by biological therapies. It cannot be predicted what specific approaches will be used; however rare cases of spontaneous remission are a proof of concept that malignancies can resolve immunologically. As a matter of physics, any cell that is molecularly distinct from other cells can in principle be identified and destroyed in vivo by technological means, albeit possibly very advanced means. In 2050, nearly a century after Richard Nixon made "the conquest of cancer a national crusade," it would be wholly remarkable for cancer to remain a major medical problem.

The eventual conquest of cancer, artery disease, and other specific diseases of aging will increasingly expose the aging process itself as a cause of morbidity. Even if one escapes named diseases of aging, the physical and cognitive declines of "healthy" aging are immense and debilitating. It has been said that a pathogen that turned healthy 20-year-olds into healthy 80-year-olds would be thought worse than AIDS [11]. Without rejuvenation of underlying systems, even diseases of aging will just keep recurring like spot fires requiring constant attention. The economic costs would be unbearable. Apart from any normative questions about how long humans should live, if medicine is to avoid therapeutic nihilism it must eventually treat intrinsic biological aging. The economic and human consequences of treating everything but aging will be too severe to ignore.

What of critical care in 2050? Along with more data about what the immune system is doing, better pharmacologic and biologic tools for managing immune function should be available. SIRS may be stoppable in its tracks. Normothermic circulatory arrest of up to 20 min may be survivable without neurological deficit by modulating the postresuscitation inflammatory cascade and other deleterious sequela of reperfusion. Survivability of longer ischemic times will allow more time for placement of cardiac arrest victims on bypass, hypothermic surgical repair of exsanguinated trauma victims, and cerebrovascular interventions.

New life support tools will be available. ECMO and dialysis can presently support cardiopulmonary and renal functions for limited periods of time. In 2050, extracorporeal replacement for all vital organs may be available. Bioartificial life support equipment may consist of integrated cardiopulmonary, renal, hepatic, endocrine, nutritional, and even hematopoietic systems. The role of critical care will increasingly be seen as providing life support for the brain to permit repair or replacement of other organ systems by regenerative medicine as needed. The affordability of such care will strongly depend on the extent to which homeostasis can be automated, as it is in living systems. The distinction between mechanical and biological life support technologies will blur.

Ultimately, the difference between sickness and health and even life and death is a difference in arrangements of atoms and molecules. The final frontier of medicine is therefore detailed control of living systems at the molecular level. While there can be many ways to wield such control, the most powerful enabling technology will be the ability to construct machines with atomic precision. This ability is called molecular nanotechnology. The emerging field of nanomedicine foresees microscopic nanorobotic devices crafted for medical applications [12, 13]. Going beyond mere pharmacologic or biologic signaling of cells, nanorobotic devices could enter cells, even necrotic cells, and perform extensive structural and molecular repairs to restore a healthy state.

In recent years detailed scaling studies have been done of some particular nanorobotic devices. These devices include the respirocyte (an artificial erythrocyte with 200 times the oxygen-carrying capacity of red cells) [14], the chromallocyte (a gene therapy vector designed to remove and replace the entire nuclear DNA content of target cells) [15], and the microbivore (an artificial phagocyte) [16]. While the capability to construct such devices lies decades or more in the future, the physical feasibility of anticipated functions can be analyzed today.

The microbivore is illustrative of the therapeutic reach of future nanomedical devices. The microbivore is an artificial phagocyte $3.4 \times 2.0 \times 2.0$ µm in dimension, consisting of 610 billion precisely arranged structural atoms (Fig. 16.5). Programmed to destroy specific pathogens, it would recognize target organisms on contact by species-specific reversible binding and then ingest them. Inside the microbivore, an ingested pathogen is to be morcellated and enzymatically digested into harmless

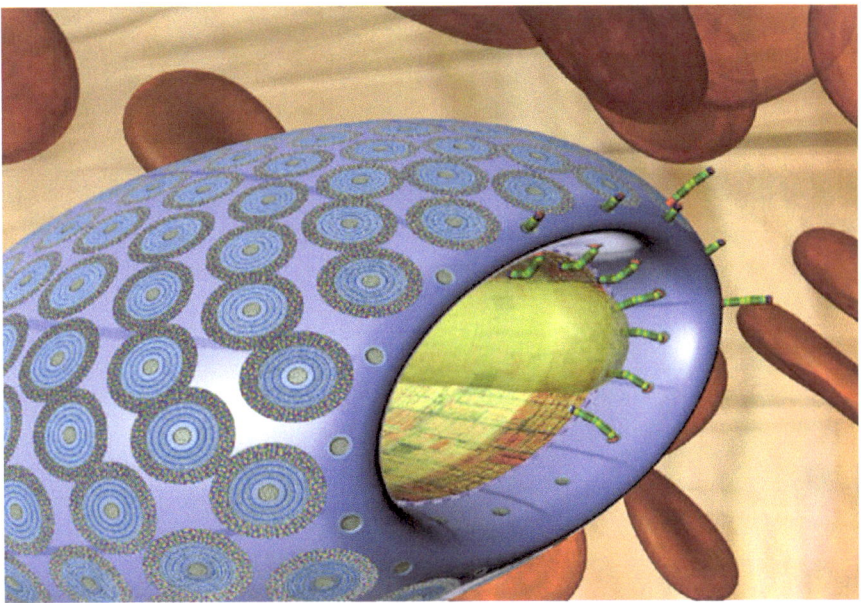

Fig. 16.5 The microbivore, a future nanomedical device for treating sepsis, shown ingesting a bacillus by extensible ciliary action. Perspective in this close-up view makes the device appear larger than red cells, although it is actually smaller (Image © 2001 Zyvex Corp. and Robert A. Freitas Jr. (http://www.rfreitas.com). Designer Robert Freitas, additional design by Forrest Bishop. All Rights Reserved)

amino acids, mononucleotides, glycerol, free fatty acids, and simple sugars which are expelled 30 seconds after ingestion. A one terabot (10^{12}) dose of microbivores has been calculated to be able to cleanse the entire blood supply of a patient infected with 100 million CFU/mL bacteria (severe septicemia) in as little as 10 minutes [16].

Devices this advanced may not exist as early as 2050, but they are in the direction that medicine is headed should technological progress continue. The future of medicine is the ability to restore and sustain life in a healthy state as we choose to define health on a molecular level. There would be many choices and time to make them.

Indefinite Lifespan

How much time? Actuarial life tables of the US Social Security Administration show the annual risk of death for a 20-year-old male to be 0.1 %, with most of the risk due to fatal injury. Taking this as a rough measure of mortality risk in a society in which aging and disease as we know them were eliminated suggests life expectancies on the order of a millennium. However, advanced technologies for repair of traumatic injuries, including repair of ischemic injury following significant periods of cardiac arrest, could reduce fatal injuries to a small subclass of what is fatal today. Future lifespans could be very long indeed.

How long would people choose to live? The New York Times in 2012 reported that given a choice between living 80, 120, or 150 years, respondents chose those lifespans at rates of 60 %, 30 %, and 10 %, respectively. Fewer than 1 % expressed interest in living indefinitely long. Remarkably, few respondents changed their answers when asked to imagine a pill that would slow biological aging by one-half.

Does the preference for 80 years of life reflect an innate biological drive? Life expectancies from young adulthood have varied throughout history and are presently increasing approximately 1 year for every 4 years that pass. It therefore seems improbable that a lifespan naturally preferred by humans would coincide with the life expectancy that happens to exist in the USA during the early twenty-first century. It seems more likely that early twenty-first-century Americans want to live as long they believe other twenty-first-century Americans will live.

There are good reasons to fear life extended beyond contemporary norms. Neither government support systems nor typical private savings are adequate to finance life much longer than standard retirement age. Nuclear families leave people socially isolated at advanced ages. Diseases of aging and aging itself cause increasing debilitation and dependence with age. Expectations of incapacitation, impoverishment, and alienation are not conducive to favorable perception of longer lives. Much more than medicine must change as lifespans increase.

Yet change will come. Lifespans will not increase by poll but by incremental additional of years to life and life to years as medicine makes people feel better at advanced ages. The resulting social changes are difficult to predict. Imagining societies with lifespans of centuries is as difficult to imagine as it would have been for our forbearers to imagine a world traversed by words and images within seconds and people within hours. Yet such a world now exists.

How will people "age" when aging is purely chronological? An obvious issue is the finite capacity of the human brain. Simple multiplication of 100 billion neurons by 1000 synapses per neuron suggests storage capacity on the order of 100 terabytes. However the brain does not store information like a hard drive until it runs out of space. The brain constantly forms and reforms connections, adding weight to what is reinforced and eventually losing that which is not. There is no time limit to such a memory mechanism. Identity becomes defined by those memories and experiences deemed important enough for reminiscence sufficient to retain them.

Some may develop expertise of unprecedented depth in fields of long-lasting passion. If 10,000 hours of practice brings perceived mastery of a field today, what if 100,000 were possible? Others may rotate through multiple careers and social environments, accumulating wide breadth of life experience. Still others may choose bohemian or hedonistic lifestyles, resources permitting. The cliché of longevity causing boredom is contrary to historical experience; as lifespans have increased so have education and career durations.

One effect of long life should be decreasing naïveté. Historically much crime and warfare has been enabled by naïve idealistic or nihilistic young men. Less naïveté could have many beneficial individual and social effects. However the flipside of naïveté is cynicism and risk aversion. Is the clichéd cynicism of old age the product of biology or the product of life experience replacing blissful ignorance?

Longer life is longer opportunity for misfortune. With longer lives, a greater proportion of the population may be affected by negative experiences with long-lasting psychological consequences. How burdens of memory are managed may determine the difference between cynicism and wisdom for chronologically aged people.

Technology sufficient to control biological aging will surely be accompanied by deep understanding of the chemistry of the brain. Understanding of "hardware" should bring with it means for ameliorating problems of "software." As just one example, to whatever extent the positive mood and outlook of youth is a consequence of brain chemistry, that chemistry could be maintained by permanent homeostatic mechanisms. Even just the ability to sleep as well as biologically young people could make a big difference in the experience of old age compared to today. Biologically healthy minds are more resilient minds.

Some will pursue modification of the brain beyond just maintenance of natural health. Direct interface of computers to efferent and sensory centers of the brain is a relatively minor modification that may become common. Electronic information available to sensory perception at the speed of thought rather than fingers could help bridge the gap between finite capacities of the brain and information retention requirements of complex careers and very long lives. Yet even this would just be "smartphone" technology with a more advanced interface. More radical changes are possible that could stretch or break the very meaning of what it is to be human. Some might argue that indefinite lifespan is itself such a change.

Indefinite lifespan is not immortality. Individuals, like communities or civilizations, are prone to evanescence. Whether by technological tampering or just the natural process of new experiences becoming more important than reminiscences of very old ones, personal identity will change over long spans of time. Rather than sudden termination, the most common form of mortality in the far future may be the continuous transformation of individuals into someone or something else.

References

1. New Semiconductors Sequence Human DNA. The State Column, July 23, 2011. http://www.thestatecolumn.com/health/new-semiconductors-sequence-human-dna.
2. Espy MJ, et al. Real-time PCR in clinical microbiology: applications for routine laboratory testing. Clin Microbiol Rev. 2006;19:165–256.
3. Dolan B. FDA approves Mobisante's smartphone ultrasound. Mobihealth news, 4 Feb 2011.
4. Harben J. 'The Doctors Is In' with RP-7 Robotic System. WWW.ARMY.MIL. Accessed 28 Sept 2007.
5. Dilger DE. FDA approves iPad, iPhone radiology app for mobile diagnoses. AppleInsider, 4 Feb 2011.
6. Murray P. Just months after Jeopardy!, Watson Wows Doctors with medical knowledge. Singularity Hub blog. 6 June 2011.
7. Krishnaraj A. Will Watson replace radiologists? Diagnostic imaging blog, 24 Feb 2011.
8. Herper M. The decline of pharamaceutical research, measured in new drugs and dollars. Forbes blog, 27 June 2011.
9. McCormick T. Innovation upturn? New medical entities/$ increasing! R&D returns blog, 29 June 2011.
10. Dong C, Goldschmidt-Clermont PJ. Endothelial progenitor cells: a promising therapeutic alternative for cardiovascular disease. J Interv Cardiol. 2007;20:93–9.
11. Personal communication with geriatrician Steven B. Harris, MD.
12. Freitas R. Nanomedicine, Vol. I: basic capabilities. Landes Bioscience, Austin, Texas; 1999.
13. Freitas R. Nanomedicine, Vol. IIA: biocompatibility. Landes Bioscience, Austin, Texas; 2003.
14. Freitas R. Exploratory design in medical nanotechnology: a mechanical artificial red cell. Artif Cells Blood Substit Immobil Biotechnol. 1998;26:411–30.
15. Freitas R. The ideal gene delivery vector: chromallocytes, cell repair nanorobots for chromosome replacement therapy. J Evol Technol. 2007;16:1–97.
16. Freitas R. Microbivores: artificial mechanical phagocytes using digest and discharge protocol. 2001. http://www.rfreitas.com/Nano/Microbivores.htm.

Afterword

Aging among critical care physicians has been written about extensively but little explored, if for no other reason than that the specialty is relatively new, and the number of practitioners near retirement age is therefore small. Most of the current literature focuses on burnout, but aging physicians in this field are confronted with something potentially more dangerous: the descent into forced or voluntary irrelevance after a professional lifetime of solving difficult problems in complex situations.

I became interested in examining the fate of the aging intensivist when it came time for me to face it. What I've done in this volume is explore the options for aging critical care physicians when they either choose to quit direct patient care, having perhaps just grown plain tired of it, or are pushed out—to make room for younger entrants, for example, or because of an inability to keep up with the changing science of critical care. Did they retire and go fishing? Teach? Become administrators? Fulfill the Peter Principle? [1]. The answers are mostly unknown, because there has not been time in this fairly young specialty for many intensivists to reach career's end.

I asked the contributors to this volume to consider some specific themes: how and why physicians entered the discipline of critical care, what critical care was like in the beginning of their careers, what their experiences were during the flood of creative innovations in critical care, and, finally, why they decided to quit (or not) and what their postretirement options were (or were not).

In relation to changes in critical care, how have intensivists evolved as they have aged? Things change in life and careers. How have they dealt with the evolution of the specialty? How have they avoided becoming irrelevant? Or have they? Retirement for critical care physicians is not the same as it is for office-based family practitioners. Aging intensivists face the frightening possibility of becoming irrelevant after decades of decisive, impactful service.

© Springer International Publishing Switzerland 2016   159
D. Crippen (ed.), *The Intensivist's Challenge: Aging and Career Growth in a High-Stress Medical Specialty*, DOI 10.1007/978-3-319-30454-0

These recollections are not geezers' personal anecdotes about the old glory days, but thoughtful revelations about the nature of aging as it applies to physicians in a high-stress occupation.

Pittsburgh, PA, USA   David Crippen, MD, FCCM

Reference

1. Peter LJ, Hull R. The Peter principle: why things always go wrong. New York: Harper Business; 2011.

Index

© Springer International Publishing Switzerland 2016
D. Crippen (ed.), *The Intensivist's Challenge: Aging and Career Growth
in a High-Stress Medical Specialty*, DOI 10.1007/978-3-319-30454-0